The health care system in Britain at the beginning of the twenty-first century is being subjected to radical rethinking. *Health Policy* examines how the NHS has developed to the point it has reached today as well as placing it in the wider context of the kinds of health care which are available to people in Britain.

It looks at key issues which have arisen in the provision of health care such as rationing, the operation of interest groups, relationships between the public, voluntary and private sectors and whether the NHS has delivered care equally to all sectors of the population.

In this second edition, the authors pay particular attention to the policy changes introduced by the Labour government following its election in 1997 and place these within a wider discussion of the concept of a primary care-led system.

Health Policy will be especially useful to readers who wish to inform themselves about what is happening in the NHS today or to deepen their understanding of current developments through an appreciation of how the health care system has evolved over the past fifty years. It includes useful summaries of key points, guides to further reading and a glossary of key terms.

Ann Wall and **Barry Owen** have published several books and articles on community health services, comparative government and the politics of health. Ann is a senior lecturer at Sheffield Hallam University, as was Barry until his early retirement in 2001.

The Gildredge Social Policy Series provides introductory textbooks to key areas of policy for the growing number of students of social policy at A level, A/S level, on GNVQ courses, in their first year at university or following a professional diploma course. Written by experienced teachers, the books are short, tightly structured texts designed to be aids to learning.

Series editor: **Pete Alcock**, Professor of Social Policy and Administration, University of Birmingham.

Also in this series:

Education Policy   Paul Trowler
Crime and Social Policy   Mike Stephens
Family Policy   Fran Wasoff and Ian Dey
Health Policy   Ann Wall and Barry Owen
Housing Policy   Jean Conway
The Environment and Social Policy   Michael Cahill
Social Work and Social Care 2nd edition   Lester Parrott

Health Policy

Second edition

Ann Wall and Barry Owen

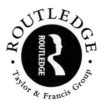

London and New York

First published 2002
by Routledge
11 New Fetter Lane, London EC4P 4EE

Simultaneously published in the USA and Canada
by Routledge
29 West 35th Street, New York, NY 10001

Routledge is an imprint of the Taylor & Francis Group

© 2002 Ann Wall and Barry Owen

Typeset in Times by M Rules
Printed and bound in Great Britain by
TJ International Ltd, Padstow, Cornwall

British Library Cataloguing in Publication Data
A catalogue record for this book is available from the British Library

Library of Congress Cataloging in Publication Data
Wall, Ann (Ann L.)
    Health policy / Ann Wall and Barry Owen. – 2nd ed.
        p.   cm. – (Gildredge social policy series)
    Includes bibliographical references and index.
    1. Health policy – Great Britain. 2. Medical care – Great
Britain. 3. Health planning – Great Britain. 4. National Health
Service (Great Britain).   I. Owen, Barry. 1943–   II. Title.
III. Series.

RA395.G7 W353 2002
362.1′0941–dc21   2001048579

ISBN 0–415–27555–5 (hbk)
ISBN 0–415–27556–3 (pbk)

To Toby, Gemma and Ben
Maggie, Simon and Kyla

Contents

Illustrations

Figures

Tables

Part I
Background

Chapter 1
Preparing the ground

OUTLINE
The years between the two world wars, and the experience of the Second World War, produced a deep desire and readiness for fundamental changes in the relationship between the State and its citizens. In the 1945 general election, in spite of the personal popularity of Winston Churchill, the Labour Party was put into power with a resounding majority with the mandate to build the Welfare State foreshadowed in the wartime Beveridge Report. This chapter focuses on the task of restructuring the system of public health care so that it satisfied new principles more generous than those of earlier times.

The importance of the Second World War

It is tempting to see the creation of the National Health Service (NHS) and the changes that it brought to the everyday lives of the citizens of the United Kingdom in a sort of 'Big Bang' scenario made up of:

- the election of the Labour Government in 1945
- the passing of the NHS Act in 1946
- the actual setting-up of the NHS on 5 July 1948.

The temptation is understandable. The Second World War was a new kind of war that involved the whole population, civil as well as military. The 1945 general election produced the first Labour Government with a solid House of Commons majority, which could allow it to enact its programme. And the new Government enacted major pieces of legislation, including the 1946 National Health Service Act. But this view is too simple in that it paints a before-and-after picture of unqualified bad turning into unqualified good.

Even before the war, there were many signs that all was not well in the relationship between the State and the mass of the population, particularly the poor, the young, the unemployed and the sick. For example, although the British Medical Association (BMA) was ever watchful for what it saw as threats to the status, pay and conditions of doctors, it had already put forward proposals aimed at widening the availability of medical care funded through national health insurance, so that coverage would extend beyond the wage earner to include the family and to provide for specialist services.

Similarly, there was widespread recognition that existing arrangements, whereby most hospitals were run by local authorities, although about a quarter were independent and voluntary, were unsatisfactory and that the two streams needed to be more closely integrated.

However, if we compare the government's view of the obligations of the State towards its citizens, in the middle/late 1930s and fifteen years later, it is clear that there had been a fundamental re-ordering of priorities. By 1950, there was a Welfare State, which included an NHS. A decade earlier, some of the bits and pieces had existed, but not enough to form a complete jigsaw. There had been, without doubt, a major change.

The origins of change

This change can be traced back to the public health legislation of 100 years before, whereby Parliament began to define a role for local authorities. There were Public Health Acts in 1848, and (following the report of the Royal Sanitary Commission) in 1872 and 1875. However, the legislation allowed measures rather than compelled them, and the response of local authorities varied widely. But the 1848 Act created the General Board of Health and the 1872 Act created sanitary authorities with the duties of appointing Medical Officers of Health and providing public health services. The growing number of public authorities operating at local level (and not just in the field of health care) needed to be rearranged into a local government system, and this, too, happened towards the end of the century. The poor state of health of British soldiers in the Boer War led, via the setting-up of the Committee on Physical

Deterioration, to the provision of school meals and school medical services early in the twentieth century and legislation was also passed relating to midwifery services.

In other words, throughout the nineteenth century, government was becoming aware of, and seeking to shape responses to, health-related problems. This often produced a reaction that, though in itself inadequate, did at least expand knowledge of the scale of the problem and then led to further measures. For example, the 1875 provision for the appointment of Medical Officers of Health turned out to be full of potential, for these officials were able, particularly within the emerging local government system, to act as champions of public health. The great reforming Liberal administration, which came into office in 1905, accelerated this process of the State assuming responsibilities towards those not best able to look after themselves. The Victorian view that it was up to individuals to stand upon their own two feet had been carrying less and less conviction, and was giving way to a more collectivist view. By early in the last century Britain may not have been ready for a Welfare State, but it was ready for Lloyd George, and 1919, after the horrors of the First World War, saw the establishment of a Ministry of Health.

Britain might eventually have established a Welfare State, and an NHS, even without the Second World War. But it would almost certainly have taken longer to arrive, and longer to establish, and the details might have been different. For example, without the experience of the wartime Emergency Medical Service, the case for taking the hospitals out of both local authority and voluntary control, and effectively 'nationalizing' them, would have appeared weaker.

The Second World War, like many wars, was an important harbinger of social change. The trauma of the First World War had been followed by disappointment. 'Homes Fit for Heroes' remained only a slogan; the reality, for many, was unemployment. But the Second World War turned out to be different from anything experienced before and its impact was even greater. Bombing of civilian targets meant that the whole population was involved. The whole of economic life had to be bent towards victory, and this involved controls on everyday life on a scale that had never before been experienced.

And there were more specific factors at work. The formation of the Coalition Government under Churchill in 1940 brought the Labour Party into the heart of government, with the Labour leader, Attlee, assuming the post of Deputy Prime Minister by 1942. Apart from what this did to public perceptions of Labour politicians, it also gave them experience of ministerial office.

The war also showed that extensive State direction of economic life was a practicable proposition. Five years' experience of a war economy showed that the argument that there were areas of activity where government was simply incapable of getting involved was groundless. And, quite apart from direct controls, 1941 saw the first budget put together along Keynesian lines, i.e. being used as a device to keep inflation down. This opened the way for budgets to be seen as more than just devices for keeping government expenditure to a minimum but, instead, as a method of guiding the economy, sometimes towards deflation and sometimes towards expansion. In other words, budgets could be used as a way of helping governments to do things rather than as a brake on their ambitions. This had further implications for the role of the Treasury, which henceforth would find it more difficult always to say no.

The Beveridge Report

The high point of this climate of change was the publication of the Beveridge Report in 1942, which was a blueprint for the future Welfare State, based on three fundamental assumptions:

- the NHS;
- family allowances;
- the maintenance of employment (Addison 1994, p. 169).

The Coalition Government was divided in its reactions to the Report. Broadly, the Labour members were in favour of acceptance at once, while the Conservatives were more hesitant, sometimes opposing its recommendations in principle. Churchill was reluctant to give firm undertakings before the war was over, preferring to wait and see what would be affordable. He was able to impose his view on the Cabinet, which in turn made Labour MPs unhappy with Labour ministers. But the widespread approval given to the Beveridge Report in the country at large could not be ignored, and by the Spring of 1943, Churchill was broadcasting promises that the war's end would see a new House of Commons legislating in a number of major areas. Although no detailed commitments were given, this was almost a promise that victory would be followed by the implementation of a great number of Beveridge's proposals.

By the end of the war it would have been close to unthinkable for the post-war government – Labour or Conservative – not to have started constructing what became known as the Welfare State, including a national system of health care. Education in the period after the war had already been taken in hand with the passing of the 1944 Education Act, and family allowances were provided even before the Labour Government took office.

Post-war negotiations with the doctors

Although it was evident that a national system of health care was necessary, there were still many details to be decided. The government had issued tentative proposals for a comprehensive health care system during the war, but these had envisaged a major role for local authorities that horrified the BMA and led to a stalemate until the 1944 White Paper *A National Health Service* got discussions going again. Even so, the BMA fought a rearguard action almost until July 1948. The leading figures in the BMA only gave in when faced with the undeniable fact that many GPs were actually signing up to the new Health Service (the consultants and their Royal Colleges had been more receptive to Aneurin Bevan's ideas from the start).

As the Labour Minister of Health, Bevan had a reputation as something of a socialist firebrand, but he was also a skilled politician, and was willing to build upon existing ideas and to negotiate. Possibly the most fundamental decision concerned what to do about the hospitals. Within a few weeks of becoming Minister of Health, Bevan decided, effectively, to nationalize them. The Emergency Medical Service during the war had shown that this was a possibility, and there had been serious concerns about the financial viability of the voluntary hospitals after the war. Bevan decided that the most effective solution would be to bring all the hospitals under the control of his Ministry. There was disagreement within Cabinet but, with the backing of Prime Minister Attlee, Bevan won the day.

The details of these disagreements and compromises can be found elsewhere (see Addison 1994, Chapter 10; Hennessy 1992; Timmins 1996; Willcocks 1967). What is more important is to note the basic shape of the system that came into being in July 1948, and the principles that it was supposed to enshrine.

The new NHS

The NHS was essentially tripartite, being composed of:

1 Hospitals
2 General medical and dental practitioners, pharmacists and opticians
3 Health care services (provided by local authorities)

See Figure 1.1.

In one sense this was an extension of what had gone before, since by 1939 there was already quite a wide range of health care available to most people. These arrangements had grown up in a rather piecemeal fashion, however, and were less than adequate in coverage, quality and geographical distribution. To some extent, then, the NHS was meant to tackle questions resulting from a lack of clarity and inefficiency. It had a practical, administrative element to it, which Klein (1995) describes as a rational paternalist approach (an approach that stretched back to Edwin Chadwick's General Board of Health exactly 100 years before).

And yet the NHS was meant to be much more than this. One of Bevan's favourite words was serenity, by which he meant peace

Hospitals	General medical and dental practitioners, pharmacists and opticians	Health care services (provided by local authorities)

Figure 1.1 The tripartite NHS

of mind and freedom from worry. It was the task of the new Service to provide serenity for all and without distinction. The 1946 Act took a particular view of health care, seeing it not as an individually-based right made real through a transaction between doctor and patient, funded via insurance. Instead, health care was established as a public good, freely available to all, an intrinsic part of a civilized society. This explains why, for example, the very wealthiest, who could easily afford to pay for private health care, were included in the scheme. They, too, were a part of society. They paid their taxes and they were also entitled to use the NHS.

The importance of taxation

People do not pay taxes solely in order to finance the services that they, individually, receive. Taxation is essentially a collective undertaking, and individuals pay in order to finance, in a general way, the activities which government undertakes for the benefit of society as a whole. The NHS was to be paid for through the tax system; this would justify the free delivery of NHS services to the population at large, whatever their tax status. These arrangements are consistent with the universal principle, which holds that the care and treatment provided by the NHS should be available to all. In other words, simply being a member of society, regardless of age or sex, or how much tax is paid, is all the qualification one needs. And again, in keeping with the spirit of the NHS, care was not to be offered on a limited basis for a restricted range of conditions; rather, the Service was aimed at the full range of medical needs.

The founding and establishment of the NHS, then, can be portrayed at two levels, the first more limited in scope, the second more fundamental and wide-ranging. At the more limited level, the 1946 Act knocked into shape and built further upon developments that had already been taking place. Setting up the NHS was a major administrative undertaking. But the detailed working-out of how the new arrangements would operate was supported by the more fundamental commitment and set of values that the new Service intended to enshrine and make real. These can be summed up as the intention that, in future, the provision of health care should be:

- universal
- comprehensive
- free at the point of delivery
- available to all who needed it.

This was meant to be a fresh start of epic proportions, and was seen as such by the general population. It is not difficult to understand the place that the NHS quickly came to occupy in the affections of society in general, which, in turn, explains the anxiety of Conservative ministers during and after the 1980s to reassure the voters that the NHS was safe in their hands.

It is easy to be caught up in the optimism of the years immediately after 1945, but dreams seldom last for ever, and it is no surprise that, the 'finest institution ever built by anybody anywhere' (Hennessy 1992, p. 144) was less than perfect. It was, after all, designed by fallible human beings. Eventually, optimism had to give way to more mundane questions about the bases on which health care should be provided, the structure of the machinery of delivery, and, most persistent of all, the cost of it. It is with these questions that the rest of this book is concerned.

Key points

- There was a wide measure of agreement, even before 1939, that improvements were needed to the existing health care system.
- The experience of the war brought about a consensus in favour of the kind of change proposed in the Beveridge Report.
- The arrangements for health care set in place in 1946, with the benefit of wartime experience, were in part a continuation and further development of what had gone before.
- There was a strong ethical component, realized through the founding principles of a health service that was universal, comprehensive, and free of charge at the point of delivery.

Guide to further reading

The period from 1945 to 1950 was an extraordinary one in British social and political history. Having won through to victory at last, the next few years were to combine much grimness and austerity in everyday life with high hopes for building a new future. This atmosphere is captured wonderfully in Peter Hennessy's (1992) *Never Again*, London: Jonathan Cape.

Paul Addison's (1994) *The Road to 1945*, London: Pimlico, reminds us that what happened in the five years after 1945 was in large part conditioned by developments during the war and, indeed, during the twenty years between the two world wars. Nicholas Timmins' (1996) *The Five Giants*, London: HarperCollins Press, is eminently readable for the same period. Finally by way of general background, the slow seeping through of everyday grimness is well conveyed in Robert Harris' (1995) novel *Enigma*, London: Hutchinson.

Concentrating more specifically on health care and the NHS, the first chapter of Rudolf Klein's (1995) *The New Politics of the NHS*, London: Longman, is both perceptive and interesting, while A.J. Willcocks' (1967) *The Creation of the National Health Service*, London: Routledge and Kegan Paul, illuminates the interactions of the various interest groups with a stake in the new undertaking.

Chapter 2

Change and development

OUTLINE

The National Health Service rapidly won the approval and affection of the British people. But the passing of time suggested that there were flaws in its design and problems in its operation. This chapter looks at these flaws and problems and at the various attempts to remedy them. Some attempted remedies were *ad hoc* and tactical, whereas others involved more fundamental reorganization. The most ambitious attempts of all came during and after the 1980s, with the introduction of general management followed by the internal market, and then, from 1999, an attempt to radically reconfigure the whole health care system.

Introduction

If the establishment of the NHS in 1948 was cause for self-congratulation, it was not long before clouds began to gather. Within five years the Guillebaud Committee had been set up to examine the dilemma of continuing to provide an adequate level of health care without, at the same time, condemning the Treasury to having to meet ever-rising costs. Over the following decades the problem refused to go away. Responses were sometimes piecemeal, aimed at a particular problem such as the need for investment in hospital building. At other times attempts were made at more fundamental remedies, either by changing structures or, particularly after 1982, by changing what went on inside the structures.

Changing the structure 1948–74

As shown in the previous chapter, provision of health care prior to the NHS had developed along the three lines of GP services, hospitals, and local authority services, and this tripartite structure continued essentially unchanged after 1948, as shown in Figure 2.1.

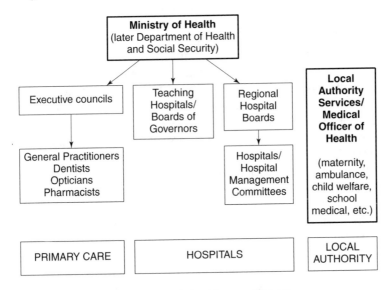

Figure 2.1 The structure of public health care, 1948–74

- *Primary care* was provided through the general practitioners (GPs) and others, who generally constituted the first port of call for the patient. They were independent contractors rather than salaried employees, and their contracts were administered by Executive Councils, whose members were appointed partly by the clinicians themselves, partly by the Ministry and partly by local authorities.
- *Secondary care* was provided by the hospitals, most of which operated within a structure of fourteen (later fifteen) regions, each with a Regional Hospital Board appointed by the Ministry. Teaching hospitals were outside this structure, operating in direct contact with the Ministry.
- *Local authorities* continued to provide a range of public and personal services, although they had lost their responsibility for hospitals.

This tripartite structure was to remain essentially unchanged until 1974, although it was apparent that there were problems with the way in which the system was functioning. The links between the three parts of the structure sometimes appeared tenuous, and when remedies were sought they were usually looked for in one or other of the three sectors rather than throughout the service as a whole.

In 1956, the Guillebaud Committee had drawn attention to a backlog of capital spending needed for new hospitals. An 'increasing gulf' was also developing between GPs in their surgeries and consultants in their hospitals (Ham 1992, p. 19). In general the first quarter century in the life of the NHS was a period of low morale among GPs, and they were slow to take advantage of Bevan's generous financial incentives for establishing health centres, so that by 1963 there were only eighteen, purpose-built centres operating in England and Wales (Allsop 1995, p. 54). On the local authority front, there was considerable variation in the range of health and welfare services provided.

These problems elicited various responses. The 1962 Hospital Plan promised £500 million for capital expenditure over the next ten years. 1963 saw the publication of *Health and Welfare*, relating to local authority services. Given, however, that local authorities enjoy their own democratic base and a measure of independence from central government, the Ministry of Health could be much less definite, so that the document was really more of a survey of the differences between authorities and a set of hopeful proposals than a plan as such. Local authority provision remained something of a disappointment to central government, in spite of the fact that the 1959 Mental Health Act implied a reduced role for hospitals and an increased role for local authorities in caring for the mentally ill. However, growing interest on the part of both GPs and local authorities led eventually to a steady growth in the number of health centres, particularly after GPs' working conditions were improved through the 1966 Family Doctor Charter.

Improvements in various areas notwithstanding, it became increasingly clear during the 1960s that an underlying problem concerned lack of integration between the different parts of the structure. It hardly needs stating that the needs of individual patients are liable to spill over between the different sectors. Some patients who begin by going to see their GP will find themselves being referred to hospital, and some of those will continue to need the assistance of local authority health services after the hospital has discharged them. Clearly, the three sectors should be working in such a way that they each support the efforts of the others in providing for the needs of patients. By contrast, the risk with a tripartite structure is wasteful duplication and poor co-ordination (which, incidentally, contributed to the fragmentation of primary care, see Chapter 9). These risks are present in many organizations, but there were features of the NHS which rendered it peculiarly susceptible to them.

The details of the tripartite structure meant that it was not under the direct control of the Ministry of Health. As we have seen, local authorities had an important role to play, and they are not just creatures of central government. Giving local government a responsibility makes central control inherently more difficult while, at the same time, creating the possibility of varied provision between different local authorities. In addition, family practitioners were independent contractors, so that if, for example, GPs chose not to be attracted by the idea of health centres, then the Ministry was limited in the pressures it could bring to bear. Thus, co-ordination by the Ministry of the three parts of the structure was always likely to be problematic. The dilemma arose not only from the fact that it was tripartite but from the actual details of the tripartism.

It fell to the Labour Government elected in 1966 to begin the process of discussion and consultation that would eventually lead to the first major reorganization of the NHS since 1948. In the attempt to secure greater unification, a first proposal was for the creation of about fifty area boards, which would be responsible for health services in their areas. A further Green Paper increased this number to ninety, with regional councils above them for planning purposes and, below or within the areas, about two hundred district committees to provide an avenue for local participation. The Conservative Government, which came into office in 1970, further developed these ideas and incorporated them into the National Health Service Act of 1973. This Act came into effect on 1 April 1974 – the same day as the new, reorganized local government system began to operate.

Public health care 1974–82

There was a wide measure of agreement within the political parties that the ideal solution to promote greater unification would be to hand over the health services to local government. However, as Klein points out, this idea, while supported in principle, was also recognized to be a political non-starter due to the continuing deep hostility of the medical profession to any notion of coming under local government control. Similarly, the proposal to transfer local authority services to the NHS was opposed by the local authorities (although they did lose their community health services). Instead, and very much as a second-best solution, the boundaries of the new Health Authorities (HAs) were aligned with those of the new local authorities (Klein 1995, p. 82), see Figure 2.2. The new innovations were:

- Family Practitioner Committees replaced Executive Councils.
- Regional Health Authorities replaced Regional Hospital Boards. Below the Regions were a new layer of Area Health Authorities, and within the larger Areas was a further layer of District Management Teams.
- Community Health Councils (CHCs) were an innovation intended to go some way towards representing the views of consumers and interest groups (see Chapter 5).

The reorganization took place at a time when great faith was placed in structural change, but structural change cannot achieve very much if the same processes simply carry over into the new structures. In the case of the NHS reorganization, the gains from greater unification were less than had been hoped for. The teaching hospitals lost their special status, their Boards of Governors, and their direct access to the Ministry, so there was some greater unification within the hospital sector. But there were now three levels below the Ministry (region, area, district), and the family practitioners still remained independent contractors separately administered.

The need for greater integration between the NHS and local government was fudged, along with Sir Keith Joseph's dream of improving management efficiency through restricting Area Health Authority appointments to those with known management ability.

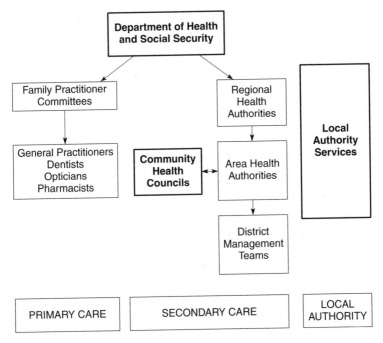

Figure 2.2   The structure of public health care, 1974–82

Faced with both the doctors and the local authorities pressing for representation, and with the practical difficulty of recruiting enough people with business experience, Joseph compromised by conceding representation to doctors and nurses as well as to local authorities. Representation for the doctors is justified by the central role that they play in the actual delivery of NHS services. However, clinical expertise is not the same thing as management ability, and one effect of this compromise was to confirm the already considerable power enjoyed by the doctors.

In a further compromise, management by those with known management ability had now given way to the idea of 'consensus management'. In practice, this turned out to mean no such thing. The management teams, which were appointed at all levels, included nurses, accountants and administrators as well as doctors, and it was hoped that one result would be to shift priorities away from acute medicine towards community health services but this did not happen. Consensus management gave a veto power to the various members of the teams, which they proved more than willing to use in defence of their own sectors. More specifically, the role of administrators continued to be seen as pre-eminently one of giving the doctors what they needed. It would take a further reorganization (Griffiths 1983) and the internal market, before managers could really begin to assert themselves against the clinicians.

Changing the structure again – 1982

The effects of the 1974 reforms were disappointing, and were soon criticized. In the meantime, however, much deeper changes were developing on the British political scene that would lead to the election of a Conservative Government in 1979 led by Margaret Thatcher. Thatcherism was to lead to changes in many areas, including the provision of health care.

The Conservatives had gone through the 1979 election campaign promising to match Labour's commitment to increased spending on the NHS. The new Secretary of State, Patrick Jenkin, was aware of problems in the NHS which the 1974 reforms had failed to resolve, but his first instinct was to continue along the path of structural change that had been followed in the past. In 1976, the Labour Government had appointed the Royal Commission on the NHS (the Merrison Commission), which reported in 1979 soon after the Conservatives came into office. The Report referred to the many achievements and successes of the NHS but nevertheless suggested improvements, including that one of the management levels below the regions should disappear, as should the Family Practitioner Committees (Royal Commission 1979). The government rejected the latter recommendation but accepted the former, so that from 1 April 1982, the areas and districts were replaced by 192 District Health Authorities. Within districts, encouragement was given to further delegation to management units, although the idea of a chief executive was rejected on the grounds that it would not work in a service which was necessarily so reliant on a wide range of professionals (see Figure 2.3). The NHS, then, went through its second re-structuring within ten years, with little hint, however, that the years to come would make 1974 and 1982 pale into insignificance.

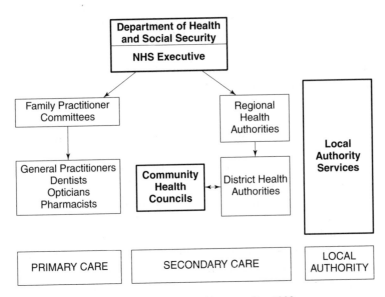

Figure 2.3 The structure of public health care, after 1982

Changing the processes – Griffiths and after

The first step down this new path was taken when Roy Griffiths, Managing Director of Sainsbury's, was asked to look at manpower in the NHS, but insisted that what really needed looking at was management. The result was the Griffiths Report in 1983 which constituted a blast against consensus management, with the now famous comment that if Florence Nightingale had been carrying her lamp through the corridors of the NHS then, she would almost certainly have been searching for the people in charge.

Griffiths called for the replacement of consensus management by general management at all levels. Administration should be replaced by management, and doctors should be encouraged to become managers (see Chapter 5). At the centre there should be a Health Services Supervisory Board responsible for setting strategy, and a Management Board responsible for actually managing the NHS. The result would be more dynamic and proactive leadership able to constantly press for improvements and monitor progress. The government accepted the Griffiths recommendations and established the NHS Management Executive under its own Chief Executive and HAs were given until the end of 1985 to appoint general managers at all levels. This went some way towards separating out policy-making and management. It institutionalized the idea that management was more than just administration, and that it had an agenda of its own within the broad strategy (and funding) set out by the politicians and officials in Whitehall. Moreover, the management function should be operational at all levels of the service.

Griffiths, then, was being put into place but it was shortly to be overtaken by a crisis relating to NHS funding. After the expiry of the three-year commitment to increased spending, attention had shifted to generating extra resources through other means. In what has been described as 'a maelstrom of initiatives' (Timmins 1996, p. 406), Derek Rayner's Efficiency Unit extended its cost-cutting scrutinies beyond Whitehall and into the NHS. Authorities were told to make efficiency savings, surplus land began to be sold off, and such management techniques as performance indicators began to be introduced. However, it was becoming more and more common for HAs to run out of money a couple of months before the end of the financial year and to respond by closing wards. By the second half of 1987, after a third consecutive Conservative general election victory, the NHS was in a state of financial crisis that regularly made media headlines. By the end of the year 4,000 beds had been closed, including some intensive care facilities for children, and the presidents of three of the Royal Colleges had issued a warning that urgent action was needed (Timmins 1996, p. 457). In January 1988, Margaret Thatcher stepped directly into the fray on *Panorama* by announcing an NHS review.

The review was conducted by a very small number of ministers, led by Thatcher, civil servants and advisers. It considered a number of possible remedies but gradually came around to the idea of a purchaser–provider split and an internal market, based on ideas which had been put forward a couple of years previously by the American health economist Alain Enthoven. The basic idea was simple. Services would be provided by hospitals and community units as self-governing Trusts, and those services would be purchased by HAs and by fundholding GPs who would control their own budgets. The providers would be in competition with one another to sell their services, while the HAs and GPs would be anxious to obtain the best value that they could for the money that they were spending. There would be, in effect, a quasi-market operating within the NHS, which would serve as the continual spur to even greater efficiency (see Figure 2.4).

Not surprisingly, the reforms ran into opposition, not least from the BMA, but the Health Minister, Kenneth Clarke found allies among the new, Griffiths-style managers who saw that the internal market could boost their position in relation to the hospital doctors. Clarke, and his successor William Waldegrave, refused pleas to soft-pedal or delay implementation. It was never intended that all GPs would become fundholders or that all hospitals and community units would become self-governing Trusts immediately; nevertheless, the reforms could have fizzled out if too few signed up for the first wave from April 1991. In the event, 57 hospitals and 1,700 GPs began operating under the internal market.

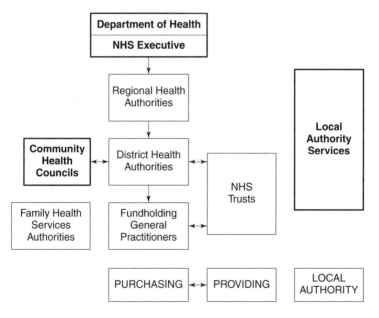

Figure 2.4 The structure of the internal market

The NHS and the internal market

In the second half of the 1990s, the NHS was still recognizable in the old, tripartite terms, with the founding principles of a comprehensive and universal service, largely free at the point of delivery. But the interrelationships between the different parts of the service had changed markedly.

The introduction of the internal market underlined the potential importance of the management function, particularly at the lower levels, where health care services are actually provided and purchased. Although, as a matter of record, general management and the internal market were not introduced as a single package, they certainly complemented one another. Arguably, the negotiating and contracting that were at the heart of the internal market needed to be driven by proactive management. At the same time, the market provided managers with the opportunity to practise their trade to the fullest extent. The growth of the internal market also led to a change and reduction in the role of the Management Executive and of the Regional Health Authorities, so that their relationship with purchasers and providers became more distant.

The result was that the most important players to emerge, at least on a short- to medium-term basis, were the HAs and the fundholding GPs, on the one hand, and the self-governing hospital and community health service Trusts, on the other. The HAs had the function of assessing the health needs of their populations and of contracting with the Trusts for the purchase of those services not already being purchased by the GP fundholders, while the fundholders purchased those services which they needed for their patients. The HAs and the fundholders, then, were the purchasers, while the Trusts provided the services for them to purchase. Outside of this there were still Directly Managed Units which had not (yet) taken on Trust status, as well as GP practices, which were not (yet) fundholders, but the intention was clearly that they would become less and less significant.

In addition, Family Health Service Authorities, descendants of the old Executive Councils and Family Practitioner Committees, were responsible for paying out the money to the contracting professions as well as for monitoring their service provision.

During the 1980s, their management role was strengthened until, in 1993, they were merged with the HAs to form Integrated Health Authorities. And, finally, the CHCs continued, rather constrained in their staffing and budgets (see Chapter 6), but still with a role to play in linking the general public to the other parts of the system (see Figure 2.5).

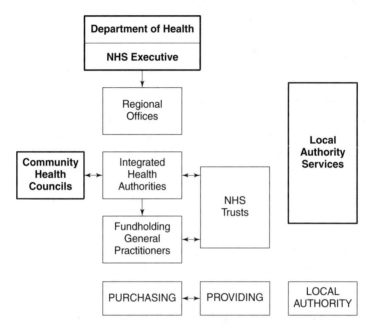

Figure 2.5 The structure of the internal market, from 1996

Subsequently there was debate about how far private sector management values, practices and techniques could be imported into the public sector (see Chapters 4 and 8). Given the popularity of the NHS, it would have been surprising if the internal market had not aroused some strong reactions. It is true that public sector organizations were established for reasons other than simply to make a profit. It is equally true that, in a democratic political setting, they (and their managers) can be subject to politically inspired constraints – to do with levels of funding, or of capital investment, or the setting of priorities – not of their own choosing. But, allowing for admitted differences, there are undeniable similarities between management in public and in private settings.

In any case, the internal market was not intended to fully replicate a private sector market. It was meant only to be a 'quasi-market'. The consumers were not individual customers, but HAs and GPs acting (and spending) on behalf of those members of the public who needed health care; the suppliers were the Trusts, competing with one another for the contracts of the consumers (Le Grand and Bartlett 1993). But if the internal market was not intended to be a real market, it was meant to replace monopoly provision with a competitive atmosphere and incentives to greater efficiency.

There had been, in effect, a change of strategy for the NHS on the part of the politicians and the policy-makers. As shown, the earlier reforms of 1974 and 1982 were mainly structural. With the introduction of general management and the internal market, however, it was the processes that go on within the structures that were being changed. By 1997, when the Labour Government published the White Paper *The New NHS, Modern and Dependable* (Department of Health 1997b), the intention was to bring some alteration to both structures and processes. Structurally, Primary Care Groups and Trusts (PCG/Ts) are compulsory groupings of GP practices. In terms of processes, while the split between purchaser (now more commonly referred to as commissioner) and provider has been retained, the emphasis has shifted from competition to collaboration, both vertical and horizontal and extending beyond the formal boundaries of the NHS (see Chapter 9).

Key points

- Concerns about costs of and operational problems within the new health care system began to emerge within a few years of its inception in 1948.
- The tripartite structure failed to operate as the seamless web of care for which health problems often called, and central control was difficult to implement.
- The structural reform in 1974 was meant to address the question of lack of coherence between the different parts of the system, although in the end it fudged the question of NHS–local

authority links while, at the same time, introducing a number of layers which added to complexity and led to the further reform of 1982.

● From the early 1980s, under the Thatcher administrations, the focus of attention began to move away from structures to the processes inside those structures.

● This led to the introduction of general management from 1983, and, towards the end of the decade, to the internal market.

● From 1997 the Labour Government introduced further changes, this time to both structures and processes.

Guide to further reading

Chris Ham's (1999) *Health Policy in Britain,* London: Macmillan, is thorough and wide-ranging over the whole field, while Rob Baggott's (1998) *Health and Health Care in Britain*, Basingstoke: St. Martin's Press, is the ideal handbook. Judith Allsop's (1995) *Health Policy and the NHS: Towards 2000*, London: Longman, approaches the subject from a variety of angles, but Chapters 1–5 are particularly pertinent to the subject matter of this chapter.

Chapter 3

The health care arena

OUTLINE
Most people in Britain receive the majority of their formal health care from the NHS. However, this is an incomplete picture. Families play an important part in determining lifestyle; informal carers provide valuable support for vulnerable kin; voluntary organizations make an important contribution; and the commercial sector plays a part in the provision, funding and supply of health care. This chapter seeks to outline these roles and to explore some of the key issues, such as the State's reliance on informal carers and voluntary organizations, the implications of the informal caring relationship for both the carers and those for whom they care; and the debate to which the recent renaissance of the voluntary and commercial sectors has given rise.

Introduction

We cannot fully understand the British NHS without recognizing the landscape of health care in which it exists. Its creation did not entail the abolition of private or voluntary provision. In addition, there remains a frequently neglected, but important, informal sector. Provision outside the NHS is particularly pertinent in the present climate in which the responsibility for meeting needs has increasingly been shifted from the State on to the family and independent sector.

The informal sector

Broadly, this can be said to comprise networks of families, neighbours, colleagues and friends. In pre-industrial days the bulk of responsibility for caring for the sick, elderly and disabled rested here and, although throughout the twentieth century there had been increasing intervention by professionals, often through the medium of the State, the everyday work of caring for dependants still takes place within the informal sector.

Families and communities

It is here that much of the control over lifestyle, now known to play a large part in determining health, lies. Cultural norms and practices with respect to diet and recreation, for example, are established within families and local communities. It is here also that the day-to-day business of shopping for and cooking food, arranging leisure activities and determining many aspects of the physical environment take place. Moreover, family and friendship networks serve to mediate between individuals and those formal services concerned with health promotion, by taking children to clinics; attending school medical inspections; encouraging other family members to attend well person clinics and to participate in screening programmes. All of this, of course, is part and parcel of what might be considered the 'normal' caring role of families.

Informal care

When the amount or type of care given goes beyond the norm (however ill-defined that norm), the term 'informal care' is applied. The first national survey of informal carers defined them as people looking after or providing some regular service for a sick, handicapped or elderly person living on their own or in another household (OPCS 1992). The survey, carried out as part of the General Household Survey, found that 4 per cent of adults were providing informal care for a dependant living in the same household (co-resident carers); 10 per cent were caring for dependants living in another household (extra-resident carers); and 19 per cent of households contained an informal carer. In total, six million adults were informal carers, meeting many of the physical, social and emotional needs of dependent people including:

- attending to matters of feeding and personal hygiene
- providing companionship
- organizing social activities
- administering medication
- performing basic nursing duties
- acting as a conduit between the user and the formal network of services (e.g. mobilizing services, arranging appointments, organizing transport).

The reasons why people become informal carers are varied. In some cases, the carer willingly takes on the role, but all too often the carer feels compelled or pressured to do so. All carers have to make personal sacrifices, particularly with respect to paid work since they are often bound to the house. Physical and emotional exhaustion, resentment, stress and a sense of exploitation, are commonly reported, among even the most willing carers (see Davey *et al.* 1995, especially Chapters 12 and 45). In other words, there are heavy economic, emotional and social costs attached to informal caring.

For recipients, informal care casts them in the role of supplicant. Abrams (1978) argued that the distinction between informal and formal care rests both on different criteria for eligibility and on rights to care. People become eligible for informal care by virtue of their social relationships, whereas eligibility for formal services is determined by bureaucratically defined criteria. With respect to rights, in the informal sector these are ill-defined and unwritten.

The nature and extent of informal caring vary considerably. At one extreme, it may involve as little as an hour or so a week; at the other, it is likely to be a full-time and onerous commitment for 'the single carer working alone in her own home carrying out, all day and every day, all the tasks akin to those of the nurse, the home help, the care assistant, and the social care manager' (Ungerson 1987, p. 154). It has been calculated that, on average, a co-resident carer spends fifty-two hours per week on caring duties and an extra-resident carer nine hours per week so that, 'if we ascribe a nominal value of £4 per hour to the work undertaken then informal carers as defined by the General Household Survey undertake work to the value of £15,599–24,041 billion per annum' (Victor 1991, p. 153).

Relationship with the formal sector

Without informal care, care in the community would be untenable for many people and formal services would be placed under even greater pressure. Equally, if informal carers are to continue to provide such extensive care they need the support of formal service providers, a situation acknowledged by Griffiths (1988). In an ideal world the two sectors would be mutually supportive, each working to its strengths in providing elderly and other vulnerable people with a 'seamless web' of care. In reality, there is overlap and interweaving of tasks, ambiguity surrounding the division of responsibility, and inadequate support from the formal to the informal sector.

Part of the reason for this is the domestic, private nature of informal caring work, which means the costs to the carers are often unseen, and consequently underestimated, by those responsible for supporting them. Another reason is that community care policies since the 1980s have been shaped by the desire of governments to control levels of public spending and justified by the contention that there is a solid core of informal care which should form the basis of all care.

> We cannot operate as if the statutory services are central providers with a few volunteers here and there to back them up . . . we should recognise that the informal sector lies at the centre with statutory services and the voluntary sector providing expertise and support.
>
> (Health Secretary Patrick Jenkin, 1980,
> quoted in Allsop 1995, p. 100)

Gender and caring

The OPCS Survey found that of the 6 million carers in Britain, 3.5 million were women. While men and women care for their spouses fairly equally, daughters are much more likely than sons to be caring for elderly parents. For children with disabilities, the mother is almost always the chief carer.

Male and female carers view their role differently. Ungerson

(1990) suggests that men are more likely to refer to love as the motive for caring and yet to talk about caring as work, using language drawn from the labour market. Gender differences are grounded in the assumption that caregiving is a normal, natural role for women. Women are more likely to be expected to become the informal carer in the first place and, when they do, gender-related assumptions in the formal services result in men being given more support than women. For example, district nurses generally expect female informal carers to cope better than males with the result that men cared for by their wives are visited less frequently than wives being cared for by their husbands (O'Keefe *et al.* 1992).

These assumptions are reinforced by structural pressures on women, particularly to do with employment. The career patterns, low pay and part-time nature of much female employment mean that, for many women, it makes more sense to take on the role of carer than to continue in employment and pay someone else to do it. There are also social pressures. Nurturing and caring are not seen simply as women's work but as a source of satisfaction and fulfilment for women, even as a defining characteristic of femininity. Thus, women experience social pressure to care for relatives and, quite possibly, stigma if they do not.

Supporting the carers

The prominence of informal caring is likely to increase in the future as the numbers requiring care increase, access to formal services is reduced and the pool of informal carers diminishes. As a result, the needs of informal carers have been increasingly recognized.

Their refusal to continue to be taken for granted (O'Keefe *et al.* 1992) prompted the launch of the New Deal for Carers in 1989 by several organizations including the Carers National Association, Kings Fund, National Schizophrenia Fellowship, Alzheimer's Disease Society and Age Concern. Part of this initiative was the formulation of *A 10 Point Plan for Carers* (O'Keefe *et al.* 1992). This raised important political questions about the carers themselves and their relationship with the formal sector. One of the most controversial points in the Plan referred to payment. There is a view that, from both the carer's and user's point of view, informal caring can, or even should, be done only for love and that financial reward would sully the relationship by clouding the motive of the carer. The counter-argument is that financial recompense for carers would provide real practical support and also recognize their important contribution. Such ambiguity helps to explain the scepticism with which initiatives such as the invalid care allowance were greeted. They could be viewed as a step towards formal support for the contribution that carers make or as a way of obtaining 'welfare on the cheap' (Baldock and Ungerson 1991).

Less controversial are the points in the Plan which relate to the belief that formal service providers should support carers rather more effectively than they have done in the past. While resources may be constrained, the views, needs and preferences of informal carers in areas such as need assessment, defining quality and information dissemination can be taken into account. This would ensure that the knowledge and expertise of informal carers are fed into the policy and decision-making process. As part of its ongoing concern that this should be the case, in 2000 the Carers National Association launched a one-year national campaign entitled A Fair Deal for Carers.

The voluntary sector

Voluntary organizations cover the spectrum from large international enterprises such as the Red Cross and UNICEF through national bodies such as Age Concern and MIND to local concerns such as the Yorkshire Association for Disabled. What they have in common is that they are non-statutory bodies, set up and run by their members rather than by government and accountable to their members rather than to the public through democratic procedures. They may be registered charities (like most of those active in the health field), registered companies, chartered bodies, or have some other legal status. Essentially, then, voluntary bodies are private organizations operating on non-commercial or social principles. They make extensive but not exclusive use of volunteers: volunteers are also to be found within the statutory sector, and substantial numbers of paid employees work within the voluntary sector.

The activities undertaken by voluntary organizations include:

- direct service provision
- raising funds
- innovating and pioneering new services
- undertaking activities where, for reasons of moral, legal or religious sensitivity, it is difficult for the State to intervene
- educating public opinion
- identifying unmet needs
- meeting minority needs
- acting in a more flexible and sensitive way than statutory bodies
- offering informed criticism of State policy
- acting as pressure groups.

In carrying out these functions, voluntary organizations depend heavily on the State for financial and other forms of support (Webb and Wistow 1982). In addition to direct grants and subsidies, those registered under the Charities Act enjoy financial benefits through the relief of tax payable on money raised; a favourable status with respect to local tax on premises; and the right to reclaim tax paid by individuals on donations given as a covenant. In total, voluntary bodies in the field of health and personal social services receive £50 million annually from the central government, as well as funding from local authorities and the NHS (Baggott 1998). In times of financial stringency, however, these funds are highly vulnerable (as are donations from the public). Moreover, even at times of high unemployment, it is not easy to recruit volunteers. Consequently, the voluntary sector tends to have unpredictable and inadequate resources, making it an unreliable alternative to State health care. Indeed, the societies themselves tend to see their role as complementary to rather than as a substitute for State provision; and most accept that the relationship is one of mutual dependence and mutual benefit, with voluntary organizations making a major contribution to health care and receiving in turn a high level of support from the government.

Historical background

The origins of many publicly-funded health services lie in the nineteenth century in the pioneering work of volunteers and voluntary organizations, most notably, health visiting; community nursing; milk banks and infant welfare clinics; hospitals; the blood transfusion service; occupational therapy; family planning; and family planning and maternity services for unmarried people. They continued to be used extensively by local authorities in the provision of community health care up to and beyond 1948 (Ottewill and Wall 1990).

The voluntary role was shaped by the volume and urgency of the social problems associated with industrialization and urbanization and by the fact that governments adopted a minimalist stance. There was, therefore, plenty of scope for voluntary effort, which was viewed as the more acceptable method of both giving and receiving help. Consequently, the nineteenth century witnessed the creation of many major organizations, some of which are still in existence today, as well as myriad smaller ones that subsequently disappeared. In the mid-nineteenth century, such was the level of activity that the Charity Organisation Society was set up to rationalize and co-ordinate their efforts. At this stage, voluntary work was associated with the middle classes, particularly women for whom it was one of the few acceptable occupations and it was very clearly founded on the principle of philanthropy (rather than mutual aid).

The voluntary sector experienced a second heyday during the inter-war years when unemployment and widespread deprivation produced high levels of social need and governments that were preoccupied with the economy. With respect to health care, voluntary organizations continued to act as a major provider of basic services such as hospitals and district nursing and to contribute significantly to the care of people with disabilities.

The creation of the Welfare State in the 1940s led some to believe that the voluntary sector would disappear. Many agreed with Professor Simey that 'the solid framework of social administration must be provided by the State, which must also carry the burden of the "mass-production" services' (Simey 1937, quoted in Wolfenden Committee 1978, p. 19). Although this proved to be a reasonably accurate description of post-war Britain, the voluntary sector did not disappear. Human need is infinite and state provision, even at its best, is never perfect. So in the period between the late 1940s and mid-1970s, which might be termed the 'golden age' of the Welfare State, despite the existence of a universal, comprehensive NHS, the voluntary sector continued to make a major contribution. For example, with respect to the care of vulnerable and inarticulate groups, such as those with physical disabilities or mental health problems, voluntary organizations were sometimes able to provide services in a more sensitive way and to articulate the views of clients in a way which statutory services seemed unable to do. Moreover, their pressure group role was well illustrated in the 1960s, when MIND and other organizations exposed the shortcomings of the NHS with regard to the care of the mentally ill. Similarly, voluntary organizations were better able to reach drug dependents living on the fringes of the law or members of sexual minorities seeking anonymity.

The voluntary sector today

The NHS still makes extensive use of voluntary endeavour both by individuals and organizations. NHS hospitals even appoint organizers of such services. The associations are virtually part of the NHS itself. They have grown well beyond the nineteenth-century paternalistic image and now employ a broader range of people such as the unemployed and newly retired. Many are high-profile, orderly, and politically active organizations, such as the National Childbirth Trust, MIND, Age Concern and the Royal National Institute for the Blind. They are often run by well-known figures regarded as authorities in their areas, consulted by governments and appearing in the media as pundits. They are professional and organize their affairs along modern managerial lines, producing mission statements and business plans; adopting new methods of fund-raising aimed at small givers; and employing marketing managers.

A number of factors have contributed to this revival. First, new needs such as those associated with HIV and AIDS; specialist areas such as terminal care; and the 'new public health' have demanded innovative responses which societies such as the Terrence Higgins Foundation, London Lighthouse, Macmillan Nurses and Public Health Alliance have been able to provide. Indeed, *Care in Action*

(DHSS 1981) encouraged the use of voluntary organizations on the grounds that they were more likely to be sensitive to new demands. Second, changing social mores have generated similar challenges with respect to mental health, the use of drugs, sex education and family planning services for young people.

Third, since the late 1970s, government has relied more explicitly on the voluntary sector in its attempts to contain public spending on health care and to limit the role of the State. Under the 1977 Act (DHSS 1977) and a circular in 1988 (DHSS 1988), HAs were obliged to collaborate with voluntary organizations, which had to be represented on certain bodies such as Joint Consultative Committees and CHCs. In discussions leading up to the reorganization of the NHS in 1982, the Secretary of State for Health expressed the view that more should be done directly by the voluntary sector, leaving the State as a safety net. The care in the community initiative was the most obvious example of this.

Moreover, after the introduction of the internal market under the NHS and Community Care Act 1990 (Department of Health 1990), the role of voluntary organizations in the context of health care changed. Some HAs, in undertaking needs assessment and service specifications as part of their purchasing (or commissioning) role, consulted voluntary organizations, and, as one of the providers of health care services, voluntary organizations were sometimes in competition with NHS Trusts. Paradoxically, this placed them in the position of being both formally consulted by statutory bodies and in competition with them. The old idea of a partnership between the public and voluntary sectors founded on collaboration gave way to contractual relationships and competition.

Predictably, the expansion of the role of the voluntary sector has had a mixed reception. Few deny the important contribution which voluntary bodies make in extending and enhancing State provision and guaranteeing a degree of diversity. However, it can be said that, with the possible exception of the pressure group role, the specific functions of voluntary bodies could, and perhaps should, be carried out by the State. Certainly, the Labour Party in opposition and others (Mishra 1990) believed that the government was absolving itself of its proper responsibilities for welfare. Moreover, there is concern that the traditional campaigning role of voluntary organizations may be marginalized as a result of the new relationships with the State.

The voluntary sector itself is concerned about its ability to cope with the greater burden and, in response to the circular which recommended that HAs engage in fund-raising among the general public, protested that such a move would impede their own fund-raising activities. As a consequence, the government published supplementary guidance stressing the importance of collaboration between the NHS and voluntary bodies in the matter of fund-raising.

Interpretations of the wider impact of the voluntary role also differ. In promoting voluntarism, that is, facilitating giving in the form of time, money or expertise on the part of individuals and groups, voluntary organizations can be said to enrich the community. Beveridge stressed the importance of the moral contribution of voluntary organizations in 'making and keeping something other than the pursuit of gain as the dominant force in society' (Beveridge 1948, p. 322, quoted in Wolfenden Committee 1978, p. 20).

Over forty years later, Kingdom wrote of the 'morally integrating force . . . [which] . . . the involvement of citizens in giving, not their money, but their time to serving the community' generates (1992, p. 115).

The more cynical interpretation, however, is that people give because they perceive some real or potential private benefit, or because they feel under pressure to do so. Furthermore, people's willingness to give, for whatever reasons, can be exploited by a government wishing to limit public expenditure and responsibility. 'There is real concern that private funds raised by charities are not merely providing optional extras but funds for core services' (Baggott 1998, p. 167).

The commercial sector

The defining characteristic of the commercial sector is that the individuals and organizations of which it consists are privately owned and controlled and operate on a profit-seeking basis.

Despite the dominance of the public sector in the British health care system since 1948, the NHS has always been obliged to embrace the commercial sector, the role of which has been diverse and complex and includes:

- provision
- funding
- supply.

Provision

All types of health care service are provided on a commercial basis outside the NHS. Hospitals, nursing homes, and clinics can be accessed through the market place and practitioners such as doctors, dentists, nurses, opticians and most paramedical professionals can treat patients privately on a fee-for-service basis. The practitioners may be working outside the NHS or combining private and NHS work as their contracts allow.

Most GPs are under contract to the NHS and have not, in fact, exercised their right to undertake private practice at the same time. By contrast, the private work of NHS consultants, although until recently relatively small scale, has always been both evident and controversial. In particular, the existence of pay beds in NHS hospitals, which has allowed consultants to treat patients privately within NHS facilities, was a matter of concern over which Barbara Castle took up the cudgels in 1976 (see Chapter 6).

The situation for pharmacists is slightly different. Although also under contract to the government, they have always sold over-the-counter medicines, cosmetics and toiletries, as well as dispensing prescriptions for the NHS. In this sense they too are part of the commercial sector, working as private individuals, seeking to make a profit. The balance between the two roles, however, has always been something of an issue and with the growth of large pharmaceutical chains such as Boots and Lloyds, the local, single-handed pharmacist has become increasingly hard-pressed and the tension between the two roles correspondingly more apparent.

As well as direct service provision, the commercial sector has had a long-standing involvement in the provision of ancillary services and, with the introduction of compulsory competitive tendering for services in 1983, this has been extended dramatically.

Funding

Approximately 15 per cent of British health care is funded privately. This is still low compared with most developed countries (USA 51 per cent, Australia 31 per cent, Italy 24 per cent: Wall 1996). Private funding is normally through the medium of insurance companies but there is also a considerable amount of direct payment from the public for low-cost treatments, non-prescription drugs, appliances and therapies, and charges for NHS goods and services such as sight and hearing tests and prescriptions. Also relevant in this context are the contributions made to charities and voluntary bodies that are active in health care. The growth of compulsory competitive tendering and introduction of the Private Finance Initiative (PFI) (due to be extended through the creation of the Local Improvement Finance Trust under the Health and Social Care Act 2001) make it harder to gauge the amount of private money going into the NHS.

Supply

With respect to supply, the NHS purchases a wide variety of goods and equipment from commercial suppliers ranging from drugs and surgical equipment to bandages and crockery.

The moving picture

Together, then, the informal, voluntary and commercial sectors contribute significantly to the promotion and maintenance of health. However, the changing relationship between these participants is shaped by wider socio-demographic, economic and political factors. For example, in the 1980s, government became concerned about what it saw as over-dependence on the State and deliberately sought to shift responsibility back to the informal sector. In principle the idea of families and neighbours playing a part in promoting health and sharing the obligation for the care of the sick may be acceptable. However, it has to be remembered that the burden is not equally shared. It falls disproportionately on the poor and on women for whom there is often little alternative. Similarly, it was the perceived funding crisis in health, together with wider concerns about public spending and an ideological preference for markets which led governments in the 1980s to promote the commercial sector as a way of reducing costs and increasing efficiency.

By the end of the 1990s, however, there was a subtle change of stance. The Labour Government sought to break down old boundaries and entered into a Concordat with the Independent Healthcare Association to set out the 'parameters for a partnership between the NHS and the private and voluntary health care providers' (Department of Health 2000, para.1.1). Nevertheless, the willingness of this sector to meet health care needs depends upon the extent to which such activities represent a sound investment with good returns. Thus, it seems probable that the role of commercial organizations will always be limited and that the State will have to continue to provide for the long-term care of the chronically sick, elderly and those with mental health problems for whom the commercial sector is least well equipped. These issues will be explored further in Chapter 8.

Key points

- Since 1948 the NHS has been the dominant but never the sole player in the health care arena. The well-established informal, voluntary and commercial sectors continued to make significant contributions which, since the 1980s, have increased.
- The renewed pressure on the informal sector reflects shifting patterns of need depending upon demographic and epidemiological trends and political ideology.
- The role of the voluntary sector in health care has been cyclical and its recent renaissance is similar in origin to that of the informal sector. Again, this sector carries certain dangers relating to insufficient funding and the possibility of the State exploiting its good offices.
- Until the 1980s the role of the commercial sector in health care

was minimal, but governments concerned about levels of public spending and seeking new ways to deal with demands on the NHS are likely to increase its role.

Guide to further reading

Chapters 3 and 4 of Linda Jones' (1994) *The Social Context of Health and Health Work*, London: Macmillan, look at health work, the family and informal care in the community. She locates her discussion in the context of a wider theoretical perspective and sociological debate surrounding family and community care policies.

Although threaded through the book rather than being confined to one chapter, Rob Baggott's (1998) *Health and Health Care in Britain*, Basingstoke: St. Martin's Press, deals comprehensively with the role of the private sector in the NHS and rehearses the major arguments surrounding it in a balanced fashion.

J. Baldock and C. Ungerson's (1991) chapter 'What d'ya want if you don't want money? – a feminist critique of paid volunteering' in M. Maclean and D. Groves (eds) *Women's Issues in Social Policy*, London: Routledge, gives a good feminist analysis of issues related to unpaid caring.

J. Kendall and M. Knapp (1996) *The Voluntary Sector in the United Kingdom*, Manchester: Manchester University Press, provide a comprehensive picture of the voluntary sector. As well as mapping its scope, the book also explores some of the substantive issues and major themes such as the changing relationship with the State. Writing in the late 1990s, the authors are able to take account of the revival of the voluntary sector and the process of formalization, which has accompanied the 'contract culture'.

Part II
The issues

Chapter 4
Resources, rationing and morality

OUTLINE
As a society, we spend enormous sums of money on public health care. Initial assumptions about cost were optimistic and today the annual budget is in excess of £50 billion. This is of growing concern, and raises questions about whether the money is well spent, whether we could achieve the same outcomes at lower cost, and whether we need to think about modifying – even abandoning – the founding principles of the NHS in favour of some form of rationing of health care.

Introduction

Health care is expensive, and becoming ever more so. This is true both from the individual standpoint and for the providers of health care. It is also true whether we measure health care expenditure in absolute terms, or adjusted for inflation, or as a proportion of total public expenditure (Baggott 1998, p. 177). The high cost of health care binds together those who consume it and those who deliver it (or, in contemporary language, commissioners and providers). It is a basic element of the health care scene, and not just in Britain; rising cost is a pressing problem in many societies.

Different countries have provided health care in different ways (Wall 1996). One option (the Beveridge model), makes health care universally available and funds it out of taxation. A second possibility (the Bismarck model), again provides for universal availability, but funds it through a compulsory insurance scheme to which employers and workers contribute. A third option (the Consumer Sovereignty model) minimizes the role of the State and leaves it to individuals to protect themselves with the health insurance that they feel they need and can afford. In Britain, after 1945, the choice was firmly in favour of the Beveridge model (see Chapter 1). From 1948, most people looked to the NHS to provide the health care they needed, although a minority continued to 'go private'. The care provided by local authorities was funded through the rates (now council tax) paid by householders (although local authorities also needed central government grants to supplement their rate incomes), while the NHS itself was directly funded by central government through taxation.

This method of funding was consistent with the basic principles behind the NHS; it was also consistent with the collectivist mood of a people who had just emerged from six years of intensive warfare. There was an assumption that once the backlog of ill health had been dealt with, then the cost of health care would fall and, thereafter, would continue at an affordable level. Consequently there was little thought of rationing health care. It was to be free at the point of use, universal and comprehensive. In fact, it was to be a living example of 'from each according to his ability, to each according to his need'.

With an undertaking as great in scope as the NHS, it would be surprising if they had got it right the first time. Adjustments were to be expected from time to time. In 1966, the Family Doctor Charter improved the pay and conditions of GPs. Then in 1977, the Resource Allocation Working Party (RAWP) formula attempted to bring about a gradual, year-on-year redistribution of resources away from those regions which appeared to be over-provided with health care facilities and in favour of those which seemed to be under-provided. But measures such as these were responses to specific problems and tactical rather than strategic.

The problem of cost runs through much of the history of the NHS. Politicians have responded by continually increasing the money spent on health care, so that its budget today is higher (in real terms) than it has ever been, yet there is evidence of a growing shortfall between actual and needed (or target) funding (Ranade 1997). The efficiency savings and the sales of real estate during the 1980s were not sufficient to avoid the funding crisis of 1987, which eventually led to *Working for Patients* (Department of Health 1989a) and the internal market.

Strategic changes had been attempted. The structural reorganizations of 1974 and 1982 (see Chapter 2) were such attempts, and were intended to address resource issues as much as organizational ones. Similarly, the introduction of general management from 1983 and then the internal market in the 1990s reflected growing concern about levels of public expenditure generally.

To a considerable extent, public health care is a victim both of its own success and that of biomedicine. A century ago there were many diseases and conditions where medical science was helpless and, in any case, popular expectations both of medicine and of State provision were less. Today medicine appears capable of answering an ever-growing proportion of our health needs, and we have come to expect it to be there when we need it. In addition, we are living longer, and thus a higher proportion of the population is coming to experience the chronic conditions associated with ageing. The question is raised whether, as a society, we can (or are willing to) continue to fund public health care in a way that is consistent with the founding values. It seems likely that, sooner or later, we will have to give some careful thought to the following issues:

- the resourcing of health care
- the allocation of resources
- the possible rationing of health care.

Resourcing health care

Resourcing generally means providing money. Organizations need different kinds of resources, such as buildings, equipment or staff, and sometimes an organization's problems are not immediately financial. In the case of health care there have been concerns about *where* functions should be located (with local authorities or with the NHS), about *structure* (the original tripartite arrangements), and about *roles* (the medical profession and the managers). In a way these concerns revolve around whether the money available is being put to best use to meet a perceived need.

Broadly, there are two approaches to financing health care. The global approach concentrates on the total amount of money provided, while a more specific approach considers whether the money available is being put to best use. Of course, the two approaches can overlap. It is possible to argue that we do not spend enough on health care and, at the same time, that what we do spend could be put to better use. For the moment, we shall concentrate on the amount of money available (the global approach) and look at whether the money spent on health care meets the need.

The global approach to funding

One problem with the global approach lies in lack of specificity. We can state how much we *do* spend, either in absolute terms or as a proportion of Gross Domestic Product (GDP), but it is difficult to know how much we *should* be spending. We can quantify the short-fall between target and actual spending but, even if we were to inject enough money to eliminate the shortfall, we would be no nearer to knowing whether we were then spending enough. Comparisons are often made with other countries, in many cases showing that we spend a smaller proportion of our GDP on health care, but such comparisons do not in themselves show that we are wrong and they are right. It is possible that our population is healthier, and thus needs less medical intervention, or that our health care delivery is more efficient, or that our administrative costs are lower. The United States spends a much higher proportion of GDP on health care than we do in Britain, but much of this is spent by individuals taking out private health insurance. Administrative costs are considerably higher in America, and few would wish to move to the American model.

In any case, it has to be appreciated that the decision on how much is to be spent is a very political one. In the past the final figure was arrived at as part of the annual Public Expenditure Survey (PES). Within a total figure for public expenditure, agreed in Cabinet, a series of bargaining meetings (known as 'bilaterals') took place between the Treasury (represented by the Chief Secretary, a senior member of the government) and the ministers from the various spending departments (Grant 1993). In these bilaterals each spending minister was – quite simply – trying to get the best result for his or her department. Depending upon the pre-vailing economic climate, this might mean securing a bigger increase in the department's expenditure total or else minimizing a reduction. It is true that the PES system was introduced in an attempt to make the overall process more rational, but the fact remains, that by the time the stage of bilaterals was reached each year, the rational element had largely given way to political bargaining. To a large extent the budget was what it was each year because that was a bit more than it had been the previous year. In other words, there was a fair bit of incrementalism – or what Lindblom (1959) called 'muddling through' – involved.

After Margaret Thatcher became Prime Minister in 1979, the emphasis was usually on reducing overall levels of expenditure – if not always in absolute terms then at least as a proportion of GDP. Thus, the annual series of bilaterals more often saw ministers trying to preserve their existing budgets than hoping to increase them. But there is a pecking order, and the health budget did well in relation to most other departments. In itself this is not surprising. The NHS enjoys widespread public support and health care is always a high profile political issue. But the (relative) good fortune of health care does not alter the fact that this resulted from a process where rationality was not the most important consideration. It can also be argued that the original decision that health care should be funded out of general taxation has served to embed it firmly in a highly political decision-making process.

The intensely political nature of health spending decisions was highlighted in the dying years of the century. The 1998 Comprehensive Spending Review, replacing PES, announced increases over three years totalling £21 billion, although the BMA later criticized the way the sums had been done and suggested that the real increase was considerably less. But this argument was overtaken in January 2000 when the Prime Minister said that increased spending on health care of 5 per cent in real terms over a five-year period would bring it up to the European average as a percentage of GDP, although it was later explained that the realization of this promise would depend upon the performance of the economy. Cutting through the arguments, however, it did appear by the turn of the century that a political decision had been taken to substantially increase the health care budget, so that for 2001–2 NHS funding was planned to be £59 billion rising to £69 billion by

2003–4. At the same time, however, the National Plan and other measures implied that the NHS would be held to closer account for its spending of the money, while financial managers within the NHS were claiming that the wide-ranging targets contained in the Plan would soak up the increased funding and more.

Allocating health care

We will now examine the second approach and try to assess how far the money spent on public health care achieves the objectives behind the spending. A simple approach to this might compare what is delivered with the founding principles of the service (free, comprehensive and universal). These seem clear and unambiguous, and have met with widespread popular approval. To re-phrase the question posed by Martin Powell (1997), we can ask 'To what extent does the NHS live up to its principles?'.

Between 1946 and 1948, the principles had to be turned into practice and made a reality. To a considerable extent, however, what the health care system has delivered has been a function of two variables. One, as discussed, is the global total of resources provided by the politicians. The other has been the clinical decisions of the medics about what treatments to prescribe for the cases that come before them. In addition, there have been public health campaigns, designed to encourage people to adjust their lifestyles (see Chapter 10). There has also been a concerted effort to even out geographical disparities in the availability of health services via RAWP.

It is clear that health care resources have not been equitably allocated between all sections of the population. The NHS has not eradicated the correlation between quality of health and social class or ethnic group (see Chapter 7). Of course, there is no way of guaranteeing that all those who need health care will actually ask for it, any more than there is a sure way of seeing that resources are never wasted on those who do not really need them. Moreover, the fact that there are health care priorities implies that, within a limited budget, those not falling into a priority group might be disadvantaged. If screening for breast cancer is a priority, then something else has to give.

In short, resources have not been – indeed, could never have been – allocated so as to ensure that provision perfectly matched need. But this is not a counsel of despair. In reality, much has been achieved. Most fundamentally, post-war arrangements removed the cash nexus between the quality of care received and the ability to pay. The effect of this can hardly be exaggerated, since it established universal entitlement. In practice, the founding principles might not have been realized to perfection, but without the abolition of the cash nexus they could hardly have been realized at all. A free service, then, was a necessary condition for an equitable allocation of health care although, on its own, it could not guarantee it.

Today health care is still largely free. Although the rise in the cost of prescriptions has outstripped the rate of inflation many times over since 1979, most people do not have to pay for them. More worrying is what Timmins refers to as bits which have 'fallen off' the edges' of the NHS, in particular optical services and dentistry which are no longer freely available (Timmins 1996, p. 505), and where, in limited areas at least, the cash nexus has been reintroduced. But we have not witnessed a large-scale desertion of public health care in favour of private. For a great many people, the NHS continues to meet most of their needs for most of their lives.

Increasing the efficiency of spending

This brings us back to the ever-increasing budget for health care. The internal market reforms were about efficiency. They were accompanied by a variety of initiatives which were intended to place greater emphasis upon achieving value for money; examples were cost-benefit analysis and the Resource Management Initiative.

Cost-benefit analysis is a management tool that seeks to calculate the costs of different courses of action and of the benefits that should flow from them. Cost-benefit analysis can be useful as a tool for illuminating different possibilities but problems arise when it is used in the public sector. In general, the usefulness of this kind of analysis depends upon the quality of the information available. More specifically, where the public sector is concerned, there has, in the past, often been either a shortage of information or a vagueness about the cost of services (Flynn 1997, p. 124). Since the 1980s, however, the position has been improving, and the introduction of such practices as competitive tendering, internal contracts, performance indicators and cost centres has obliged public sector organizations to become more cost conscious. In the NHS in particular, the period during and since the 1980s has seen a veritable epidemic of data collection, including financial data (Allsop 1995), so that statisticians came to be among the key players.

The Resource Management Initiative, introduced in 1986, relied heavily on the collection and analysis of reliable data, so as to provide a bank of information about the cost and effectiveness of services and activities (Baggott 1998). The intention was that this would allow clinicians to assume greater responsibility for how they spent their budgets. Not surprisingly, perhaps, doctors were often less than enthusiastic about what they sometimes perceived as an exercise in (or, at least, a prelude to) cost-cutting. There was insufficient appreciation that, as well as data collection, changes in attitudes were also needed (Hunter 1993).

Measures such as these set a pattern for subsequent governments faced with the difficulties of controlling a budget for a service where demand is liable to keep on increasing, and where actual spending is in large part the result of myriad decisions being taken by professionals who are cloaked in clinical discretion and who do not see it as part of their job to cut costs. Later measures, for example, the move towards a primary care-led NHS (see Chapter 9), while not directly intended to *reduce* health care spending, have evidenced a continuing concern with health outcomes.

Rationing health care

At first glance, rationing does not appear to sit easily with the founding principles. It is easy to see how it offends against comprehensiveness and universality. Even if health care remains free, rationed care implies that is limited in some way, and it seems to open up a Pandora's box of unpleasant possibilities for the future. Nor does it help much to talk, instead, about prioritizing. As we have already remarked, giving a higher priority to some (whether social groups or medical conditions) implies giving a lower priority to others. Prioritizing, then, might only be a veiled word for rationing. It can come as something of a surprise, then, to learn that rationing has long been practised in the field of health care. The facts are simple. As already stated, health care is expensive, and yet the budget is limited. If the budget is not large enough to allow all who need treatment to receive it (within a reasonable period of time), then *de facto* rationing exists, if only through the mechanism of waiting lists.

It can even be argued that rationing is not so out of place in the NHS as we might at first think. It was pointed out in Chapter 1 that, as well as the idealism, the NHS also stands as an example of rational paternalism. It was designed to provide people with what they needed, and this would not necessarily be the same thing as what they wanted. What people needed would be decided, essentially, by the medical profession. There was no guarantee that individual patients would leave their GPs with a bottle of pills; they might, instead, be told to take more exercise. Similarly, and at a more general level, it is the medical profession that has set the main patterns of health care availability. Screening for cervical cancer is offered because clinicians believe that it is detectable and treatable at an early stage. Allsop cites a study looking at the selection of patients for renal dialysis, which implied the existence of a favoured group (aged between 15 and 45, otherwise healthy and married with children) who were more likely than others to be offered dialysis (Allsop 1995). Furthermore, the fact that 'Cinderella groups' (such as the mentally ill) have existed is yet more evidence of *de facto* rationing.

In other words, if we see the term rationing as a reflection of the reality of a system that can only call upon limited (albeit considerable) resources, and which allocates those resources as a result of medical rather than popular decisions, then its existence becomes more understandable. Rationing becomes not so much a betrayal of principles as an imperfection in the system.

By the 1990s a different kind of rationing had moved up the agenda, partly as a result of the growing importance of management, and partly as a result of the financial disciplines introduced by the internal market. Thus, there was a more open acceptance

that the resources allocated to the health care system were insufficient to allow it to do all that it was capable of doing, and a greater
readiness to think about the possible bases for allocating (and, by
extension, for not allocating) those resources. Baggott (1998), for
example, claims that the new rationing was more explicit than the
old.

Lessons from Oregon

Possibly the most overt step in this direction occurred not in this
country but in Oregon, USA. The objective was to include a
greater number of low income individuals and families within
Medicaid provision, but the *quid pro quo* was that the range of
medical care offered would have to be limited (Baggott 1998,
Chapter 3). Two features of the Oregon project are particularly
worth noting. First, although cost-benefit studies were used in
drawing up a list of treatments, members of the public were also
consulted (by telephone). Second, it was proposed to withdraw
some treatments (e.g. of some cancers) where only a small percentage of those treated were likely to survive beyond a certain
period after treatment. Public consultation raises the interesting
question of whose voice should carry most weight in the event of
disagreement between the public and the medical profession.
Health care provision in this country has been largely based on the
assumption that the expert knows best, and the traditional relationship between doctor and patient has not been one of equality.
However, if patients are to be thought of more as customers, then
it is presumably logical to pay more attention to their demands.
And yet, ascertaining those demands might be a problem, particularly if the public are being asked for their views on which
treatments might be excluded. Somebody who has never suffered
from, say, bronchitis might well give a different answer from a
chronic sufferer, and it would be difficult to know which view
should carry the most weight.

    There are, as well, objections to the blanket element of the
Oregon approach since, as Klein points out, it ignores the fact that
individuals are different, even in their illnesses (1995, p. 245). For
example, the Oregon proposal to cease providing treatment for

cancers with a poor prognosis ignores the likelihood that, generalized prognosis notwithstanding, some sufferers – albeit only a few – would have benefited from treatment.

Alternative calculations

An alternative to the blanket approach has been to attempt calculations in individual cases of the benefit, or improvement to quality of life, which treatment is likely to deliver. One technique has been the Quality Adjusted Life Year (QALY) formula. By applying a formula which builds in the likely survival period as well as an attempted measurement of the degree of improvement after treatment, together with the cost of treatment, it becomes possible to say which treatment is more cost-effective, whether between patients with different conditions or different patients with the same condition (Baggott 1998). Thus, spending, say, £5,000 to effect a minor improvement to the quality of life of an elderly person is less cost-effective than spending the same amount to give a much improved life quality to a younger person. Not surprisingly, clinicians themselves often feel unhappy with this sort of approach, since it conflicts deeply with the medical ethic and seems to reduce questions of life and death, distress and comfort, to economic calculations.

In the health care system of today, information and techniques are available that make rationing a more practicable proposition than ever before. Indeed, the NHS is already some way down this path. Medical audit, evidence-based medicine, and the National Institute for Clinical Excellence (NICE) are not in themselves rationing devices, but they do add to the stock of information which would be relevant to a rationing process. And, since its remit was extended to include the NHS, the Audit Commission has undertaken well over forty investigations, covering such diverse topics as GP prescribing practices, improving Accident and Emergency services, and measuring management costs.

At the present time, some rationing does happen, for example, through the mechanism of waiting lists, or through charges if they have a deterrent effect. Other rationing takes place when doctors decide not to proceed with treatment because, in their opinion, little good would come of it. Occasionally rationing comes more out into the open, when an HA decides not to purchase treatment, but these cases are likely to have been influenced by medical opinion (for example, a decision to discontinue ear grommets in cases of glue ear). There are, as well, management tools that can help to clarify at least the economics of these kinds of decisions. And yet, at the end of the day receiving treatment can be a lottery, varying between authorities and between doctors (Macdonald 1996). The HAs are responsible for purchasing health care on behalf of their populations, and so it is the HAs that are often the targets for criticism, especially when a particular case is taken up by the media. For their part, HAs often feel that rationing decisions have been forced on them by shortage of funds. Thus, at the end of the day, it comes down to money, and money for the commissioners comes from the government. Unless we argue that the NHS is becoming steadily more wasteful then, sooner or later, the politicians will have to face up to the dilemma caused by limited supply coupled with limitless demand.

Managing demand

The White Paper *The New NHS* (Department of Health 1997b) announced the introduction of NHS Direct, a telephone help and advice line staffed by nurses. Three pilots started in March 1998, with national coverage planned for 2000. If this is successful it could result in members of the public playing a greater part in the management of their own ill health episodes, in many cases not needing much more in the way of further NHS involvement. Looked at optimistically it could result in better management of demand for NHS services for those conditions which often need little more than good professional advice, in which case resources could be freed up to be concentrated more where they are really needed (Pencheon 1998). However, there is still much about the new service that remains to be finalized. It holds out the prospect of a degree of patient empowerment, but it needs a public less wedded to the idea of being able to pop into their GP surgeries. There is also, of course, the risk of media headlining the first time a nurse on the end of a telephone misjudges a situation. But, at the least, the NHS Direct idea might be an early sign of a revision of the traditional paternalist doctor–patient relationship. On the other hand, it could turn out to be another example of disguised rationing.

Key points

● The rising cost of health care has been a matter of growing concern in Britain and elsewhere.

● Responses in Britain have been partial, and sometimes palliative, without significantly alleviating the problem.

● It is difficult to know whether we spend too much or too little on health care. Deciding how much to spend is a political process that is not inherently rational. Similarly, at a global level we cannot be confident that resources are actually allocated so as best to meet the health care needs of the population.

● Increasingly, questions of efficiency have come to be emphasized, and measuring techniques originating in the discipline of economics have been employed.

● Slowly, there has developed a greater willingness to admit that some rationing of health care already takes place, albeit relatively unsystematically. However, we appear to be still a long way from adopting rationing as a formal policy response to the problem of ever-rising cost.

Guide to further reading

Rob Baggott, once again, is a reliable companion to this chapter, as is Rudolf Klein. For a general background to changing perceptions of the public sector as a whole, see Norman Flynn's (1997) *Public Sector Management*, London: Prentice-Hall/Harvester Wheatsheaf, particularly Chapters 1–4.

For a more specific examination of the issues which can arise where finite resources meet potentially infinite demand it is worth looking at Chris Ham's (1998b) *Tragic Choices in Health Care* London: King's Fund.

Questions relating to assessing and judging the record of the NHS in delivering health care, including possibilities for rationing, are addressed in Martin Powell's (1997) *Evaluating the National Health Service*, Buckingham: Open University Press, particularly Chapters 5–8, as well as in David Hunter's (1993) *Desperately Seeking Solutions* Harlow: Longman. In addition, the *British Medical Journal* has published a number of articles in recent years on the subject of rationing, e.g., Bill New (1996) 'Education and debate: the rationing agenda in the NHS', vol. 312, no. 7046, p. 22.

Taking a wider view, Angela Coulter's and Chris Ham's (2000) *The Global Challenge of Health Care Rationing* Milton Keynes: Open University Press, illustrates that resourcing problems are not confined to the United Kingdom.

Chapter 5

Interest groups in health care

OUTLINE

The public health care system is huge and complex. In addition to its three basic divisions (hospitals, primary care services, local authority services), it is made up of hundreds of smaller organizations, and it is home to major groupings of players. From a human resources viewpoint these players collectively populate the system, but their interests do not always coincide and they often approach health care questions with different considerations in mind. From the start clinicians have played an indispensable part; more recently they have had to learn to work side-by-side with a new breed of manager; more recently still there have been moves in the direction of patient empowerment. This chapter looks at some of the issues raised by this shifting picture of group dynamics within health care.

Introduction

Organizations are not simple things. Behind the formal picture, as depicted by an organization chart, lies the reality of the informal organization – the way things actually get done – and the difference between the two can be variable. A unitary perspective, which sees the different parts of the organization all working together, pulling in the same direction and dedicated to the same goals, is an unrealistic model. A pluralist view, however, accepts that differences exist *within* organizations with frequent contests played out through the interactions of different groups within the organization.

The larger the organization, and the more varied its functions, the more true is the pluralist model. In the case of health care, the undertaking is so huge that it is questionable whether it should be seen as a single organization. There is a health care system, certainly, but it is made up of hundreds of organizations, from

PCG/Ts and GP practices to HAs to hospitals and Trusts to the NHS Executive, local authorities and the voluntary and private sectors (see Chapter 3). Each of these constitutes a pluralist system in itself, which come together to form the much larger system. Additionally, there are cross-cutting links providing elements of common interest in the overall system. These cross the boundaries between different organizations, so as to provide what we might call sectors. PCG/Ts might share common concerns that are not felt by hospital Trusts; clinicians in a hospital might feel more common ground with clinicians in other hospitals than with the managers in their own hospital. Managers in NHS Trusts might empathize with their counterparts in the private health sector. When one takes all this into account, the picture becomes very complex indeed.

Ever since its establishment the NHS has stood high in public esteem, and yet it appears that it is never satisfied. Those engaged in providing health care appear always to be demanding more resources, and it is not difficult for them to back up their demands with arguments centring on the cost of research, new techniques, advances just over the horizon, or the needs of an ageing population. And the media stand ever ready to report bad news about waiting lists or refusals of treatment on grounds of expense. Health care is a very political area. Disagreement and compromise, negotiation and bargaining were present at its birth, and they have never gone away.

Pressure groups and the NHS

The health care system provides a home, or at least a focal point, for many interest groups. Such groups and their activities are at the heart of the pluralist model.

Since 1948, there have been few people who have never come into contact with some part or other of the NHS. It has played a very large part in our post-war social history, and it is not surprising that there are pressure groups whose areas of concern bring them into regular contact with the health care system. Such groups range from the British Limbless Ex-Serviceman's Association to MIND and SCOPE. They lie outside the strict boundaries of the system, and do not devote their entire attention and resources to influencing it. Their activities often bring them into contact with, while trying to influence, those with responsibilities for the delivery of health care. Sometimes this activity will be directed at the highest, policy-making levels; at others it will concern some aspect of local provision.

In addition to these groups outside the NHS, there are others that operate inside the system. These are the different groups of employees, each seeking to bend the system towards the direction that it believes to be desirable. It is to these groups that we now turn our attention, specifically:

- doctors
- nurses
- managers
- citizens and patients.

Doctors

Academic sociologists debate about which groups in society should be labelled professionals. Nurses, social workers and teachers, for example, have been described as belonging to 'semi-professions' (Etzioni 1969). But there is little disagreement that doctors belong to a profession. The professions are set apart by certain defining characteristics:

- their members will have been educated in a body of specialized knowledge;
- professionals are employed to apply their knowledge and skills;
- the skill of the members of the profession is recognized by the possession of a professional qualification, either instead of or in addition to a university degree;
- the knowledge needed to obtain this qualification is controlled and defined by a governing body such as the General Medical Council.

In this way professions can be, to a considerable degree, self-regulating concerning who is allowed to join and the degree of knowledge and skill which they must demonstrate in order to do so and it is quite common for the governing body to concern itself, not only with the technical knowledge and skill of the profession's members, but also with their ethical behaviour. There is no doubt that 'medicine has most of the features commonly associated with a profession' (Baggott 1998, p. 39). Furthermore, membership of the profession is necessary before the individual can practise as a doctor within the NHS (hence the seriousness of being 'struck off'). What is more, State involvement in the definition of who is entitled to be seen as a 'proper doctor' long pre-dates the NHS, having been established through the Medical Act of 1858 (Bynum 1994). The Act did not outlaw other approaches to health care, but it did place scientific medicine on something of a pedestal compared to, for example, homeopathy or herbalism. If the Act did not guarantee eventual victory to scientific medicine, it allowed it to define the terms of the debate about the best approaches to health care (Weatherall 1996). Scientific medicine was also helped by developments in medical science itself, so that, as time went on, it seemed increasingly to actually work. By the end of the nineteenth century we can legitimately talk about the existence of a medical profession. Admission to and continued membership of the profession were largely controlled by the profession itself, and the approach to health care in which its members were educated and trained was that of scientific medicine. During the twentieth century these essential features of medical professionalism have remained largely intact, being reinforced by the central role in the provision of health care given to scientific medicine by the NHS.

Willcocks (1967) has pointed out that the group that secured most out of the negotiations about the post-war NHS was the medical profession. This is hardly surprising. Without the doctors there would not have been an NHS, and they were able to secure much of what they wanted in terms of representation on administrative bodies, freedom from local government control and from the threat of a salaried service. The hospitals (especially the teaching hospitals) were the palaces in the new service, and within the palaces the consultants sat on the thrones.

This, in turn, affected the ethos of health care. Doctors have been largely educated into the scientific, biomedical approach which tends to focus on individual ill-health episodes. Symptoms are observed, leading to diagnosis and treatment and, hopefully, cure. It has been remarked that the NHS is really a National Sickness Service, concerned with us only when we are sick but less interested while we are still well. In other words, scientific biomedicine emphasizes cure more than prevention, individual symptoms more than social factors, and these emphases have largely determined our approach to health care. It is, after all, doctors who define and determine what constitutes ill health and, by extension, what constitutes health. Further, it is the doctors who are uniquely qualified to decide on the appropriate treatment for the cases that come before them.

The suggestion, then, is that the medical profession has not only performed its immediate task – the treatment of illness – but that, in addition, it has been able to determine the kind of health care which is available to us. The elected politicians might decide the broad parameters and set the global funding levels, but below this their influence has been extremely limited. What the health care system has actually done, on a daily, monthly, yearly basis, has been the result of the daily, monthly, yearly activities of the medical profession.

It is a further feature of professions that their members often have considerable discretion in how they operate. Professionals expect to be allowed to get on with their jobs according to their own best judgement and in ways approved by the profession itself, and if they are subject to review or direction it is likely to be by their peers. This can mean that professionals and general managers or even members of other professions within the organization are uneasy associates, with each seeing the others as blinkered and unco-operative. This has been the case in health care no less than in other areas where professionals are employed. In particular, politicians and the Treasury, in their concern with ever rising levels of expenditure, have found the medical profession unwilling to count the cost, as well as being uneasy about using cost-benefit analysis techniques in relation to patient treatment (see Chapters 4 and 6). Doctors have tended to see it as their responsibility to provide and prescribe the best possible treatment for their patients, regardless of cost. Many feel that they did not go through the long years of training just to be turned into accountants, and this unwillingness to compromise in the pursuit of savings, taken together with their central role in the delivery of health care, has added to the difficulties ministers have experienced in trying to mould the NHS to their political will.

Divisions in the medical profession

Of course, 'the medical profession' is a general term, and covers a variety of specialisms. In the nineteenth century medical professionals were either surgeons, physicians or apothecaries (what we now call GPs); today the number of specialisms runs into dozens, including psychiatry, obstetrics, gynaecology, rheumatology and many more. Some specialists, such as geriatricians, tend to be more concerned with chronic than with acute medicine; some, such as epidemiologists, will have more interest in the public health side of medicine; others, such as oncologists, might be just as interested in research as in treatment. Some doctors work in hospitals, some in research institutions, others in general practice surgeries or health centres. Not surprisingly, the profession is not always united in what it wants.

Within the profession greater esteem has in the past gone to hospital medicine, with community medicine and general practice suffering by comparison. And even within hospital medicine some specialisms, such as surgery, have had more glamour about them than, say, geriatrics or psychiatry. The position of GPs improved after the bitter negotiations that led to the Family Doctor Charter in 1966, but it was the introduction of fundholding practice in the 1990s (along with demographic and epidemiological changes) which really strengthened their hand. Subsequently the idea of a primary care-led health service opened up the possibility of a considerable shift of power within the medical profession. GP practices have been brought together in PCG/Ts and given an enhanced role, and although there is still a tendency on the part of hospital doctors to view GPs as the medical second division, it is a view that is probably approaching its sell-by date. However, internal divisions such as these are unsurprising, and the things that unite the different specialisms remain stronger than those that divide them.

Nurses

Nurses form an interesting contrast to doctors. If there is little doubt that doctors, in their many guises and specialisms, form a profession, there is more room for argument in the case of nurses. If nurses are seen as little better than doctors' helpers – making the beds and taking blood pressures so as to free up the doctors for the more important tasks – then it is difficult to describe them as a profession. Indeed, it remains true that the clinical side of nursing consists to a considerable extent in carrying out procedures and giving treatment decided by doctors.

If, on the other hand, nurses are seen more as collaborators with doctors, bringing to patient care their own body of knowledge and skills, allied to but distinguishable from those of the doctors, then nurses' claims to being members of a profession become easier to accept. Such a view would justify the existence of the United Kingdom Central Council for Nursing, Midwifery and Health Visiting, and moves to increase the number of graduate nurses. In July 1999 the government published *Making A Difference* (Department of Health 1999), proposing the post of nurse consultant in hospitals and an improved career ladder. In the primary sector, too, the introduction of NHS Direct, nurse practitioners and some nurse-led Personal Medical Services (PMS) contracts offer enhanced clinical opportunities.

In practice there is room for a considerable amount of variation in the working relationship between doctor and nurse, and that between newly-qualified junior doctor and experienced nurse might not be the same as the one between experienced consultant and a nurse new to the wards (Hughes 1988). It is also arguable that nurses subscribe to values which, while not alien to those of doctors, are at least distinguishable; that, whereas doctors are concerned with cure, nurses are in the business of care.

The picture becomes less clear as we move away from clinical questions and into the business of keeping things moving. Doctors rely on nursing staff to keep the machinery running smoothly. One writer has remarked that nurses 'see themselves as having a managerial function within a hospital' and that 'nurse managers see themselves as the legitimate and rightful heirs to senior posts in the management structure' (Fox 1992, p. 110). While managerialism, from the 1980s, represented an opportunity for nurses, it was one which Klein (1995) believes that they never fully grasped. The future for nursing staff looks brighter than it has for some considerable time past. Management posts are still available while, in addition, an enhanced clinical role is becoming more feasible. These features might go some way towards addressing continuing recruitment and retention problems.

Managers

We have already remarked that much of what is actually done in health care terms is the product of clinical decisions taken by doctors and that doctors rely on nursing staff to keep the whole operation moving along. Further, this takes place in the context of a value system, which places quality of treatment and care in a central place. And yet the 1980s saw the introduction of general management at all levels of the NHS, in a radical attempt to bring the system under closer control and to make it respond, at least in part, to other values. The message was that the private sector had much to teach public organizations, about cost efficiency and value for money, about how things should be managed. It was said that management 'is the key subsystem in the organizational system. It spans the entire organization and is the vital force that links all other subsystems' (Kast and Rosenzweig 1985, p. 5). Hannagan believed that 'managers are the people responsible for helping organizations to achieve their objectives' (1995, p. 4). This was along the lines of what Sir Roy Griffiths had in mind when he called for a structure of general management to run through the whole NHS (DHSS 1983).

The kind of management envisaged by the writers referred to above is positive, vital and central to the organization. It shows what Peters and Waterman called 'a bias for action' (1982). As self-confident players with their own agenda, there is a good chance that such managers will come into conflict with other groups in the organization if those others do not share the management vision. In the case of health care organizations, this is likely to mean the medical profession.

In the past, clinical knowledge was usually met with deference, and the discretion to prescribe the best available treatment was central to the system. Administrators in the NHS might have complained that doctors did not understand their difficulties, but they rarely questioned the idea that their job was to give the doctors what they asked for. If there was any idea of a clinical–administrative partnership, it was one where the administrators were very much the junior partners. In turn, this made it very difficult to exert effective control over the sum total of clinical activity once the broad sums of money had been allocated by the politicians. Certainly, administrators did not see it as part of their function to control the doctors.

By contrast, Griffiths (DHSS 1983) was in no doubt that the clinicians had to adjust to the real world where funds were not limitless, where economy and efficiency mattered, and where clinical activity could be judged in terms of cost-effectiveness. In order to achieve this, Griffiths proposed that the responsibility for actually running (or managing) the NHS should be taken away from the DHSS and given to a new NHS Management Executive (since renamed the NHS Executive) headed by a Chief Executive, while, at the same time, units at every level would be headed by a general manager or a chief executive. In this way managerialism and a managerialist culture would be firmly installed throughout the whole service.

Managers would be expected to be flexible and to exercise discretion and imagination in the achievement of their goals, but the NHS would be given leadership. Nor was this type of management to be anti-clinician. Indeed, it was hoped that the clinicians would accept that the use of clinical resources carried with it a responsibility for the management of those resources. Management budgeting, by turning clinicians into budget-holders, was meant to encourage them to become more aware of the larger budgetary picture and to accept greater responsibility for what they did with their own budgets.

The introduction of general management created a range of possible relationships between managers and clinicians. At one extreme, the doctors could simply give in, and allow the managers to institute whatever they liked in the way of performance measurements, monitoring and target-setting. At the other, the doctors could totally refuse to co-operate, knowing that their knowledge and skills were, in the last analysis, indispensable, and hope in this way to neutralize any management initiatives. In practice, neither extreme position was likely, and the reality varied from place to place. In general, however, the introduction of general management was less than totally successful. Managers themselves were often enthusiastic, but the officials in the DHSS effectively reined them in by showering them with directives and priorities, which mostly obliged them to concentrate on short-term cost-cutting and budget-balancing (Ranade 1997). Clinicians were frequently suspicious, and there was little the managers could do to counter this. Managers could and did have an impact, but it stopped short of the medical profession, so that, as one consultant remarked 'management stops at the consulting room door' (quoted in Wistow 1992). A deadlock developed between managers and medics, which needed some additional factor if it was to be broken. The publication of the White Paper *Working for Patients* in 1989, and the passing of the National Health Service and Community Care Act the following year, provided just such a catalyst by introducing a new feature that appeared to cry out for managerial skills and expertise – the internal market.

In short, if the doctors were unwilling to manage the internal market, then the managers would do it for them. It constituted the new high ground, territory which the managers claimed to be qualified to occupy. In primary care, too, fundholding practices were increasingly employing practice managers, while since 1999, in PCG/Ts, the chief executive has emerged as a central player.

Citizens and patients

The system of public health care established in 1948 continues to enjoy widespread public approval. But this is not to say that, having been established, it was then to operate in a democratic fashion, any more than were the nationalized mines or railways. In one sense it was democratic in that there was, responsible for running it, a minister accountable to the elected House of Commons. In another, less formalized sense, too, it was democratic in that it continued to enjoy considerable general support. But in its day-to-day operations there was little democracy in the way the NHS went about its business.

This might seem surprising, given the centrality to people's lives of the matters that were the concern of the NHS. The business of the NHS was sickness and pain, and birth, life and death, and these things are far more important to most individuals than whether interest rates rise or fall or whether the balance of payments is in surplus or deficit. And yet, from the start, the opportunities for the public to make known their wishes about the kind of health care available to them were very limited. Perhaps few people wished to make suggestions. But the fact remains that, had they wished to do so, then the avenues open to them were few.

In fact, we should not be surprised that this was the case, since it is of a part with the rationalist and paternalist approach to which we referred in Chapter 1. The NHS was set up for the people, just as the whole, post-war Welfare State was set up for them. Both were created, from altruistic motives, to meet needs. The needs having been identified by Beveridge, the details could be filled in by experts, and this was nowhere more true than in the case of health care, where there was a whole army of experts ready to supply the details.

None of this is to deny the altruism or the ethical dimension involved; instead, it is simply to point out that the public were to be catered for as subjects rather than as participating citizens. But it did mean that the role of individual patients was a passive one; once they had walked into the local surgery or through the consultant's doorway they would believe what they were told and do as they were told.

Empowering patients

Over the years concerns were expressed about the lack of any democratic input, particularly in the light of the declining role of local authorities after 1974. With respect to individual complaints, the terms of reference of the Parliamentary Commissioner for Administration (Ombudsman) were extended to include complaints of NHS maladministration in 1973. Complaints procedures were modified as a result of the recommendations of the Davies Committee (DHSS 1973) in 1973. A step (but a fairly modest step) in the direction of consulting the users was taken with the establishment of Community Health Councils (CHCs) in 1974. These had the role of safeguarding the public's interests, but, with little in the way of powers, staff or funds with which to fulfil that role (see Chapter 6), and in 2001 legislation was put before Parliament which included the abolition of CHCs.

In 1983, Griffiths still felt that the public needed to be given more information and that the new breed of manager needed to make more deliberate efforts to find out what the public wanted (DHSS 1983). However, if this raised the prospect of managers assuming the mantle of champions of the people, it has to be tempered with the realization that the new managers still had the task of establishing themselves while simultaneously coping with the directives being fired at them from the centre. Being a champion was fairly low down on the typical manager's list of priorities.

The introduction of the internal market in the 1990s may have given the impression that patients were being empowered, but in practice it was the HAs and fundholding GPs who were the purchasers, amounting to a new form of rational paternalism. Even if it was true that 'money follows the patient', it was equally true that the patient followed the contract. This still did not amount to direct empowerment of the public; it was, at best, empowerment of GPs as representatives of the public.

But what patients could expect was codified and made more specific in the 1990s through the medium of the Patient's Charter. Charterism, beginning with the Citizen's Charter in 1991, has been described as the 'policy embodiment of consumerism within public sector reform' (Falconer 1996, p. 191). This might appear to be claiming too much, especially when we remember that the charters contained little new in the way of legally enforceable rights, but we should also remember that the move to charters had strong prime ministerial backing from John Major. This is not to say that charters had the effect of overturning the traditional relationship between the citizen and the State. In the case of the Patient's Charter, the long-standing view that the clinician knows best remained strong.

In 1993 complaints procedures were re-examined by the Wilson Committee (Department of Health 1994) and as a result were simplified, but since 1997 a somewhat different approach – sometimes labelled 'dipstick democracy' – has been adopted, including the use of focus groups, patient forums, and patient advocates (intended to replace CHCs). Nevertheless, the public have never been seen as consumers in any private sector marketing sense, freely able to take their custom to another shop, nor have they been genuinely empowered as active citizens. Even against a background of growing disillusionment with the medical profession and an increased media appetite for reporting medical scandals, the government response was to set up the National Clinical Assessment Authority. This is a centralized monitoring body more in line with old notions of political accountability than consumer empowerment.

Changing relationships within the NHS

The NHS continues to rest upon deep public support, and the medical profession is still highly esteemed. Nevertheless, some changes in the relationships between different groupings within health care are now becoming clear. If the medical profession, cloaked with clinical autonomy, still stands on a pedestal, its position there is no longer unchallenged. The internal market was much more than mere exhortation and doctors were unable to ignore its requirements and procedures. Even the most reluctant medics were obliged to accept its presence, as they have more recently been obliged to accept the collaborative impulses of the *new* NHS.

In crude terms, then, the medical profession has become less powerful, while nurses have seen their power increase and the managers have found themselves more able to pursue their own agenda. Neither managers nor nurses any longer see themselves just as the medics' handmaidens, and the medics are obliged to listen to what both have to say. Although moves to empower the public have been limited and piecemeal, doctors can no longer dictate to their patients as they once could.

Key points

- The public health care system exhibits considerable organizational complexity.

- Within this complexity the system houses different groups of stakeholders, most notably clinicians, managers, and patients.

- At one time the doctors operated in something close to absolute power, with other groups occupying distinctly inferior positions, although the professional relationship between doctors and nurses has been fluid.

- More recently the role of management has been strengthened, in ways often unwelcome to clinicians.

- As managers have become more confident, and as the internal market increased the importance of the management function, so the two groups of clinicians and managers had to begin to define a new way of working together.

- Managerialism also changed perceptions of those who use the health care system. The paternalism that infused the NHS in its earlier years has become less appropriate, although there are still considerable obstacles in the way of genuine consumer empowerment.

Guide to further reading

Roy Porter's (1997) *The Greatest Benefit to Mankind*, London: HarperCollins, traces the history of medicine and medics over the past 2,500 years, but is especially interesting in its second half, where it deals with the emergence of medicine as a science in the nineteenth and twentieth centuries. Similarly, Bynum's (1994) *Science and the Practice of Medicine in the Nineteenth Century*, Cambridge: Cambridge University Press, helps us to understand how, through its claim to be scientific, medicine and those who practised it were able to establish their professional dominance in the field of health care delivery. More generally, Jonathan Gathorne-Hardy's (1984) *Doctors*, London: Weidenfeld and Nicolson, adopts a fly-on-the-wall approach to (pre-fundholding) general practice which is more descriptive than analytical, but interesting, nonetheless.

Much more recently, medics have had to contend with challenges to their position from the emerging profession of management. This is looked at in Chapters 3 and 4 of Gabe *et al.* (1991) *The Sociology of the Health Service*, London: Routledge, and in Chapter 6 of Wendy Ranade's (1997) *A Future for the NHS? Health Care for the Millennium*, London: Longman, while Chapter 5 of Nicholas Fox's (1992) *The Social Meaning of Surgery*, Oxford: Oxford University Press, concentrates on the management of surgical routines and procedures. Annabelle Mark and Hilary Scott (1992), in Leslie Willcocks and Jenny Harrow's (eds) *Rediscovering Public Services Management*, London: McGraw-Hill, analyse NHS management in some detail from a very theoretical standpoint.

Martin Joseph's (1994) *Sociology for Nursing and Health Care*, Cambridge: Polity Press, looks at doctor–patient relationships (fairly briefly) in Chapter 4, and Chapter 12 of Judith Allsop's (1984) *Health Policy and the NHS*, London: Longman, examines the opportunities for users to 'exercise their voice'. Consumerism, which is supposed to be a part of the new management, is examined by Hunter and Harrison in Chapter 6 of Iliffe and Munro (1997) *Healthy Choices*, London: Lawrence and Wishart, and Joseph Jacob, in Chapter 9 of McKevitt and Lawton's (1996) *Public Sector Management*, London: Sage Publications, forecasts a busy and prosperous future for lawyers and accountants as 'significant players in the administration of medical practice'.

Chapter 6

Managerialism, cultures and control

OUTLINE
The statist conception of the public sector, in the ascendant after 1945, gave way to one where public and private are seen as less distinct and where, more specifically, the public sector has been expected to learn from the private. In the health care field this change has been seen with the embedding of a managerialist culture. This chapter examines some of the questions raised by this change of direction, and considers the possibility that it might, after all, be misconceived.

Introduction

By the second half of the twentieth century the State was taking an interest in many more aspects of national life than ever before. This meant that the public sector had become not just larger but more complex as well. Today around five million people – over 10 per cent of the workforce – are employed in the public sector and nearly one in five public sector employees works in the NHS.

The 25–30 years after 1945 have been talked about in terms of a consensus, a wide measure of agreement about the role of government, or the State, and the extent to which it could or should intervene. This consensus largely held until the economic crises of the 1970s. Whichever party had been in office after 1974 would have found itself battered by financial storms, it happened to be Labour, and so it was the Conservative Party, led by Margaret Thatcher, which benefited at the general election of 1979. It was under Thatcher's premiership that the post-war consensus, and with it the public–private interface, was re-examined – a process which has continued since. The belief that the public sector could, to the benefit of all, be made to behave more like the private sector resulted in a variety of measures during and after the 1980s, and the delivery of health care was not untouched by such measures.

Public and private

Gerald Vinten reminds us that, 'There has never been an absolute distinction between public sector and private sector, nor has a "pure" public or "pure" private sector ever existed' (1992, p. 4). Nevertheless, there were surely differences between them. Public and private sector organizations have existed for different reasons, with different sources of finance, different clienteles, different owners, different measures of success or failure and, flowing out of all this, different cultures (see Chapter 8).

If we imagine a continuum, with health care being exclusively a public sector concern at one end, and exclusively a private sector concern at the other, then it is true that, from 1948, Britain was placed towards the public sector end of the line. But it was never at the extreme end point. Most people chose to use the NHS but a portion of the population preferred private medicine and contributory insurance schemes existed to make this possible.

Private and public health care systems have therefore existed side by side with links between them. At a general level the fortunes of private medicine have varied as a function of the economic climate. In times of recession some subscribers to private health care have withdrawn or else downgraded their cover. At other times, when the NHS was perceived to be in crisis and so less reliable, private health care has seemed to some to be more attractive. More specifically, the NHS allowed a degree of private health care within its own four walls right from the start. Consultants could choose to be part-time, which meant that they could supplement their NHS salaries with income from private practice. There was provision for pay beds in NHS hospitals as well as for consultants to use NHS facilities in treating their private patients. After 1979, Conservative Governments introduced measures which, while not designed to harm the NHS, encouraged both the growth of the private sector and the degree of interdependence between private and public medicine (Higgins 1988). From 1997, Labour Governments, far from reversing these measures, further elaborated them in the NHS Plan and the Concordat (Department of Health 2000).

To return to the continuum mentioned earlier, the growth and diversification of the private health sector in recent years do imply a shift away from the public end, but it is only a shift, and health care for most people, for most of the time, continues to be publicly provided. Trust status for hospitals, for example, does not mean entering the private sector. But it does mean behaving differently, and the more significant change is summed up in the various attempts to oblige the different organizations within the NHS, while still remaining within the public sector, to operate in line with private sector imperatives. General management, working within the internal market framework, constituted the biggest initiative but there were others. From 1983, compulsory competitive tendering for ancillary hospital services such as laundry and catering was intended to introduce market disciplines. The Health and Medicines Act of 1988 gave HAs opportunities for income generation and, since 1993, the PFI has allowed and invited private sector investment in NHS capital projects. The public and the private health care sectors, existing in pure isolation from one another since 1948, have in recent years become more mixed together. Having said this, however, we should also remark that the intention was for the public sector to learn from the private and to become accustomed to a process of marketization.

Arguably, public health care today is neither one thing nor the other. It exists for the same reasons for which it was first established, it still has the same clientele and it is still subject to ultimate control by elected politicians (rather than by shareholders and a Board of Directors). But, although its finances still come overwhelmingly from public taxation, the way in which money travels around within the system is now more closely tied in with performance. Thus, measurement of success or failure now has an undeniably stronger financial component. It is no longer enough simply to treat the sick; this now needs to be done with one eye on the budget. In other words, rather than just providing health care, the system is now enjoined to manage that provision with economy and efficiency, and this has come as something of a culture shock to those schooled in the ideologies of curing and caring.

The cultural impact

Organizations have their own cultures, and one writer has described the effect of culture as being to teach the members of the organization 'the way we do things here' (Hannagan 1995, p. 224). In fact, a culture is something of a rag-bag, a collection of ideas, values, norms and assumptions, but the reason it matters is because it affects behaviour, and gives rise to a certain consistency and coherence in values and attitudes.

Certainly, management writers think it worthwhile to talk about organizations' cultures. Morgan (1986) cites Robert Presthus, who suggests that we live in an organizational society, and that organizations are mini-societies that have their own distinctive patterns of culture and sub-culture. Many such writers argue that the culture can be manipulated so as to make it better serve the needs of the organization, and even those who stress the difficulties involved in such manipulation nevertheless admit the importance of organizational culture.

The delivery of health care has gone through changes that run so deeply that the fit between culture (particularly that of the clinicians) and practice has been called into question. This is a problem for those who believe that public health care must learn from and adapt to a changing environment. The difficulty lies in getting the cultural side of things to stand still long enough for us to examine it. This is a common problem in the social sciences, where students cannot isolate and alter different variables as can, say, the chemist in the laboratory, and it is made worse by the nebulous nature of culture.

However, in the case of health care there are organizations that can make the task a little easier. Hospitals are central to the delivery of much of health care. They are the places where the biomedical approach is seen most clearly; indeed, it has been in hospitals that many of the advances in biomedicine have taken place, since they have functioned in effect as medical laboratories. Up to a point, a large hospital has a life of its own. It is open twenty-four hours a day and, for those admitted as in-patients, it can (for a while) become the central focus of their lives. Joseph (1994, p. 26) has suggested that a hospital – along with prisons, seminaries and the army – can usefully be seen as a 'total institution . . . where a large number of people come together and where they are relatively cut off from the wider society'. And it is institutions such as these that tend to exhibit a strong culture.

For many years after 1948 the clinical culture was dominant in hospitals. The doctors (assisted by the nurses) were the people who actually delivered the product, in the forms of diagnosis, treatment and (it was hoped) cure. The introduction of a managerial culture resulted in two sets of values co-existing within the hospital. Neither could ignore the other. The managers had the backing of the politicians plus a growing confidence in themselves as they sought to move towards the status of a profession. At the same time, the doctors continued to be the ones who had the medical training, although now they were obliged to apply their knowledge and skills within a more entrepreneurial framework. In the last analysis, without the doctors the managers would have had nothing to manage; on the other hand, the doctors needed the managers to work the machinery. Some sort of coming together of the two sets of values, of the two cultures, needed to occur. The personification of this was the clinician-turned-manager, and there were examples of this with the post of Clinical Director. But it was too much to expect the medical profession as a whole to be converted to the culture of managerialism.

When consensus management was introduced in 1974 it was intended to be a new process of team-based decision-making which would work through bargaining and compromise and which would, incidentally, produce a shift of emphasis away from acute, hospital medicine. In practice it failed. It was part of a reform package that allowed the same processes as before to continue. Consensus management gave the various participants a power of veto; it merely produced delays and did nothing to change the culture but, rather, endorsed the prevailing power of the clinical veto (see Chapter 2).

Inducing cultural change takes time and yet culture is not static. It can adjust when reality changes. The 1974 reforms were not sufficiently deep to upset the prevailing culture. By contrast, Griffiths-style general management, combined with marketization, amounted to an earthquake that altered the landscape of the NHS.

Many medical professionals might not have liked it but, this time, they could not continue to act as if nothing had happened, particularly since they now needed the managers to make the new system work. This is not to say that a revised culture, to which both medics and managers can happily subscribe, immediately emerged. But the political reality changed, and some medics (for example, some Clinical Directors and some fundholding GPs) positively welcomed this. In crude power politics terms, if the managers stood their ground, and if they continued to receive political backing, then there was the possibility of a new managerial/medical culture emerging.

Ownership, control and access

The decisions about the delivery of health care which were enshrined in the NHS Act of 1946 meant that, in one sense, the NHS belonged to us all. Health care was seen as being what economists call a 'merit good ' – something which the market, left to itself, cannot be relied upon to supply in sufficient quantity or quality, but which is held to be so desirable that government intervenes to ensure its supply. The founding principles, and the method of financing (out of general taxation), meant that all were 'members' of the NHS, even if some chose not to use it.

But the term 'public ownership' can be a misleading euphemism. At no point could a member of the public point to a hospital, or even a single bed, and say, 'This belongs to me'. Instead, public ownership really means – in keeping with the merit good concept – something operated on behalf of the public by a public organization. Public ownership, then, is somewhat removed from ownership in any generally understood sense of the term, and has more to do with politics than with law. Furthermore, the same approach applied to questions of control, so that, just as the public could not be said really to own health care, nor did they have any meaningful rights of control over it. There is, in fact, quite a neat logic discernible here. Ownership generally carries with it connotations of control. The person who owns a thing is likely to control its use, and inability to control use implies absence of (or, at least, restrictions on) ownership.

This is in keeping with the rational paternalist approach of the early NHS. The public were to be beneficiaries rather than owners. Health care was for them, and it would be delivered to them, but the details were settled by politicians, officials and the medical profession, and there was little by way of democracy in the new system. Hospital Management Committees and Executive Councils and then, after 1974, the various HAs, were composed in part of lay members either appointed or approved by the minister, and in part of nominees of professional medical groups such as consultants and GPs, together with some members drawn from local authorities. At best this was a heavily diluted form of representation of local interests; indeed, one commentator implied that it was only a 'pretence that appointed members represented local communities' (Allsop 1995, p. 244), which in any case was replaced from 1990 by a more straight-forward commitment to a business ethic. After 1990, the governing bodies of HAs and Trusts would be most akin to private sector Boards of Directors, with some of the members coming from senior levels within the organization and the rest being appointed from outside for their business skills and acumen.

Such a shift had already been foreshadowed in the 1974 reforms, when it had been hoped to appoint lay members for their managerial ability. The hope had not been realized then. Nevertheless, it had been accompanied by a view that, if HAs were to have a primarily managerial orientation, then they should not be expected to fulfil simultaneously a representative function. And so CHCs were created to meet this need.

Community Health Councils

At first glance CHCs might appear to have had an impressive part to play. They might not have said much about ownership, but they appeared to be relevant to questions of control and access. They had their existence from statute and were independent of the management structure. They had the right to be consulted on local health service developments and, where they raised objections, to delay the implementation of proposed changes. They also had the duty of advising and helping individual complainants. They carried out a variety of roles from patients' champion to watchdog for local interests to information and communication channel. They could set their own priorities for action, sometimes based upon their own local opinion surveys.

And yet their impact since they were established was limited and, while they may have had some influence at the local level, it is more difficult to identify a sustained impact in terms of national health policy. Arguably, they were under-staffed and under-funded. A typical CHC office only had two or three full-time staff, while the volunteers making up the council were likely to be mostly drawn from among the retired population. Public meetings were sparsely attended, except when the occasional high-profile issue was being considered, and this suggested that the CHCs could not arm themselves with much in the way of public support.

Writing in 1979, Garner concluded that 'The capacity of CHCs to be dynamic is certainly limited' (1979, p. 152), and this continued despite other initiatives aimed at enhancing patient input (see Chapter 5). Barnes and Cox (1997) suggested that, at the same time that recent developments in health service management had increased the importance of CHCs, so too there had been an increased demand for their services. They had become busier, but the increased calls on their help had not been matched by increased resources. Even in the consumerist 1990s Barnes and Cox concluded that whereas CHCs would continue to have a role to play, it remained questionable whether they were able to play that role to the full. Baggott (1998, p.250) refers to a need to clarify their role, and the Labour Government in 2001 proposed their abolition – a proposal which, perhaps surprisingly, gave rise to some considerable opposition. It would appear that the weaknesses pointed up by Garner in 1979 have yet to be resolved.

Measurement: aiming at the wrong target?

The embedding of a managerialist culture carried with it an imperative to measure and quantify, but it is arguable that policy-makers came to place too much emphasis on efficiency and not enough on effectiveness. This emphasis was reflected in the 1980s with an undue focus on 'value for money' (VFM). It was Thatcher's conviction that VFM was best achieved in the market-place. Hence, so the logic went, if you were to import the market-place into the public sector, then along with it would come VFM. VFM was generally held to consist in the 'three Es' of economy, efficiency and effectiveness (to which some would have wished to add, particularly in the context of the public sector, a fourth 'E' – equity). Economy and efficiency were relatively easy to deal with, since they were essentially monetary and thus quantifiable. At the simplest level, economy was to do with inputs of money, whereas efficiency looked at the outputs side of the equation and meant doing more than before but with the same money. Thus, in principle, one could take measurements and say that economy, or efficiency (or both) had increased.

The problem arose with effectiveness, which is concerned with the extent to which an organization – whether the whole NHS or an individual part – achieves its goals. Measuring effectiveness is difficult where, as is often the case in the public sector, an organization has numerous and complex goals, or where the goals are difficult to specify with any great precision. For example, should the effectiveness of the health care system be measured by the overall state of health of the population or by the proportion of sick people who are cured? The temptation might be to count people as cured, or at least as treated, when they are sent home from the hospital or when they leave the surgery with a bottle of tablets. Munro (Iliffe and Munro 1997, p. 68) refers to this as 'finished consultant episode (FCE) inflation'. Indeed, this has happened because the contracts and service agreements that lie at the heart of the system are based on performance targets of this kind, and those delivering health care are under pressure to meet these targets. In short, there is the possibility that the clinical ethic will give way to meeting the targets in the contract. If this were to be the case, it would amount to adjusting the figures so as to give the appearance of meeting quantity targets, but at the expense of quality of patient care. However, Munro (ibid., 1997) argues that clinical effectiveness is an intrinsic part (indeed, a prerequisite) of VFM in health care, and that improvements in effectiveness would necessarily include improved efficiency. It is true that attempts are being made to measure and improve clinical effectiveness, for example with 'evidence-based medicine' (ibid., p. 56) and the introduction of NICE and clinical governance, but there are still tensions between the existence of clinical discretion and the imperative to measure.

In terms of cultural change it can certainly be argued that a logjam was broken through the processes of marketization. Those responsible for delivering health care have had to take more account of the world outside their surgeries and hospitals than used to be the case. GPs are no longer the poor relations and public health promotion is firmly on the agenda. While clinical autonomy has been largely preserved, the medical profession can no longer ignore the wider management agenda.

But a management culture has been expensive and the costs of running the system have risen as a proportion of overall cost. The assumption that the cost of management will be more than offset by savings elsewhere remains not proven.

In the last analysis, the case for a managerialist culture rests upon the assumption that it will lead to improved VFM. The risk is that quantifiable improvements will be presented in evidence to disguise a falling-away in quality of care.

Key points

- By the middle of the twentieth century the public sector as a whole was large and complex, reflecting an assumption of responsibilities by the State which, in its turn, rested upon a new post-war consensus.

- In the late 1970s this consensus came under attack. The public sector was portrayed as wasteful and inefficient and compared unfavourably to the private sector.

- Public sector organizations, including those of the NHS, have been encouraged to learn from and imitate the private sector.

- The reforms involved have gone so deep as to require changes of culture in the organizations affected. In the NHS the clinical culture has been confronted by a managerialist culture which it cannot ignore.

- CHCs might have been expected to play an increased part in representing the general public. However, their ability to do so, as well as their future role, remain uncertain.

- It would be unjust to dismiss managerialism as having failed. Nevertheless, there is room for debate about how far considerations of VFM are appropriate to the health care setting. Arguably, what is really needed is a greater concentration on clinical effectiveness.

Guide to further reading

Chapter 2 of Le Grand and Bartlett's (1993) *Quasi-Markets and Social Policy*, London: Macmillan, looks at the theory of quasi-markets, while Ian Tilley's (1993) *Managing the Internal Market*, London: Paul Chapman Publishing, considers a wide range of aspects at both general and more detailed levels. But Chapter 5 of Wendy Ranade's (1997) *A Future for the NHS? Health Care for the Millennium*, London: Longman, is the best short, sharp, but effective treatment of a topic where so much ink has already been used, while Chapter 8 of Baggott's (1998) *Health and Health Care in Britain*, Basingstoke: St. Martin's Press, is, as ever, solidly reliable.

Chapter 7

Inequality in health and health care

OUTLINE
Members of minority groups have inferior health, poor access to health care services and poorer employment opportunities in the NHS. The pattern of inequality and disadvantage reflects that of wider society. There are powerful moral, legal and economic arguments in favour of change. This chapter seeks to examine the nature, causes and impact of inequalities and to assess measures to promote equality.

Introduction

Inequality exists both among users and providers of health services. The patterns of inequality reflect those in wider society. A founding value of the NHS was equality of access to health care for all British citizens but, although widely accepted, proved one of the hardest to apply; indeed, inequalities appear to have widened rather than narrowed. We have also come to recognize differential access to health which has little to do with the NHS, and there is growing unease about the disadvantage experienced by certain groups with respect to employment.

The purpose of this chapter is to examine the nature and causes of inequality from the perspective of both service users and providers. These two standpoints are related. If women, members of minority ethnic groups and other disadvantaged groups are not adequately represented among NHS decision-makers, then their needs and preferences are less likely to be reflected in services. In fact, the manner in which services are designed and delivered tends to reflect the norms, values and interests of white, middle-class males. We will also examine some of the initiatives designed to secure better access to health, health care and career development for disadvantaged groups.

The main focus of the chapter is on inequalities associated with class, gender and race but it is important not to lose sight of other less 'visible' groups who may also be vulnerable to discrimination on the grounds of age or sexual orientation.

Minority groups and discrimination

In understanding why some groups are disadvantaged, the concept of 'minority' can be used. This may be a numerical minority (e.g. black people in Britain), but it can be a social minority, denoting not the size of the group but its lack of status and power, as with women. The reasons why some groups are accorded a subordinate position in society are complex and linked to the human tendency to generalize and make judgements:

- Most judgements are made without full and adequate information; they are premature, pre-judgements. This is the literal meaning of the word prejudice, meaning unfounded and generalized views about others.
- Judgements are often based on stereotypes, that is, standardized images fashioned by the wider socio-political context.

Discrimination

The process of prejudging and stereotyping is a way of reaching a conclusion quickly despite not being in possession of all the facts. Important decisions may be based on these dubious snap judgements, which reflect stereotypes rather than careful consideration of the evidence. In other words, irrelevant criteria such as gender or race may have an undue influence. This is the essence of discrimination and where it happens consistently and systematically, it can generate rules, regulations and procedures that work consistently in favour of some groups and to the disadvantage of others.

Discrimination can be of two types: direct and indirect. Direct discrimination means treating members of one group less favourably than those of another, for example, allowing a middle-class woman to give birth at home but pressuring a working-class woman to go into hospital; deciding to send a white nurse on a management training course rather than an equally well qualified black colleague. Indirect discrimination occurs when a condition is applied in such a way that the proportion of people from one group who can comply with it is considerably smaller than the proportion of another group. For example, healthy eating advice is easier to follow where the family budget is adequate; a decision to hold a breakfast meeting is likely to generate more problems for women with children than for women without children or for men.

The case for equalizing opportunities

There are, of course, strong moral objections to discrimination. In terms of natural justice, people should be treated fairly and equitably. Arguably, the NHS, as a large, visible public body with an explicit ethical dimension to its work, should serve as a role model for other service organizations in providing an equitable service and in widening opportunities for and promoting the interests of minority groups.

However, there are now additional arguments, particularly relating to employment. First, since the mid-1970s there has been a growing body of legislation, rules and initiatives, both national and European, which outlaw certain forms of discriminatory behaviour. Thus, in order to stay within the law, the NHS is obliged to take the issue of equal opportunities seriously.

Second, the ever more urgent need to maximize the use of its resources has driven much of the NHS's development. With almost a million employees (3.5 per cent of the UK workforce), the NHS is the largest employer in the country. However, familiar and well-established demographic trends mean fewer young people entering the labour market. Changing family patterns and the evolving role of women mean that more women work outside the home and more people combine employment with domestic duties. The emergence of new skills and professions has been a feature of the NHS as has the impact of information technology. These factors, taken together with the more explicit emphasis on competition, have changed the face of NHS employment and mean that employers can ill afford to waste or under-use talent, particularly in the light of current problems relating to the recruitment and retention of nurses (Buchan 2000).

Ross and Schneider suggest that:

> [while] the ethical case stands up . . . it is the economic case that will win the argument . . . in the tight labour market for skills, employers have a strong incentive to ensure that they make their selection decisions based on merit and create an environment in which all individuals can develop.
>
> (1992, p. xxi)

Third, the NHS is more likely to be demonstrably effective with a diverse workforce which reflects the community it serves and is, therefore, sensitive to the needs and preferences of patients and better able to work in partnership with them. Moreover, as the organizations of the NHS work more autonomously and have to enter into contracts and other working relationships with independent bodies, so their diversity and political correctness will serve as an attraction to such bodies.

Class

The advent of health services free at the point of use in 1948 removed the price barrier that had restricted access for many poorer people (see Chapter 1). Unfortunately, this did not secure the expected equal access to services and did nothing to reverse the persistent class gradients in health status.

One aspect of the problem is that the poor tend to live in areas where services are less adequate. Even by the 1970s, in the industrial areas of the North of England and Wales:

- there were fewer hospital beds per head
- hospitals tended to be older
- doctor–patient ratios were less favourable
- there were fewer specialized medical staff
- facilities were of poorer quality.

Predictably, health indicators, such as the infant mortality rate, varied in line with this. Attempts to remedy the situation such as controlling the distribution of GPs had failed, and the system of funding the NHS tended to perpetuate geographic inequalities. RAWP (1976) introduced a formula designed to ensure that resources were allocated according to health need rather than historical accident and, with its later variants, it did go some way to rectifying geographic inequalities. However, it occurred at a time when resource constraints had begun to bite, so it was inevitably based on the principle of shifting resources from those areas of the country deemed to be over-resourced to those deemed to be under-resourced; a process which caused resentment in the areas which lost out through the formula.

Further research in the 1980s found that there were still quite startling geographic variations in the level of provision (Jones 1994). In 1997, a study comparing life expectancy in all 105 HAs demonstrated that the gap between the most affluent and the poorest areas of the country had widened over the past ten years (Raleigh and Kiri 1997).

The Black Report

In 1977 the Labour Government set up a working group on inequalities in health, chaired by Douglas Black (DHSS 1980). Its remit was to review information about differences in health status between the social classes, to consider possible causes and the policy implications and to suggest further research.

The report, presented to a Conservative Government in 1980, demonstrated that, while mortality rates for men and women aged over 35 in social classes I and II had fallen, those for people in social classes IV and V were the same or marginally worse. Ill health, it seemed, is indisputably linked to poverty. The Report met with a chilly response from the government, but media interest and the publication of *Inequalities in Health* (Townsend and Davidson 1982) assured it gained wide attention.

The resounding message from Black was that to tackle ill health we must tackle poverty so he recommended raising child benefits, introducing non-means tested free milk for babies, more health education, better recreational facilities in inner cities, national health goals and anti-smoking measures. But its recommendations were rejected by the government on the grounds of cost, which was estimated at £2 billion. The government was not prepared to tackle the issue of poverty. Its policies had, in fact, resulted in more poverty as increased numbers of people came to depend on low pay and benefits. Inevitably, therefore, a report that found that poverty also damaged health and that the health problems of the poor could not be laid solely at the door of the NHS was unlikely to find favour.

In spite of the inaction, Black can be said to have been a seminal influence in the health debate, drawing attention to the fact that medical care was only one (and not necessarily the best or most efficient) way of influencing health. It revived the idea (neglected since the nineteenth century) that health improvements could be achieved by concentrating on housing and income maintenance. Almost ten years later the message of the Black Report was re-affirmed (Acheson 1988).

In 1987 the publication of *The Health Divide* by Whitehead confirmed Black's findings and broadened the debate, demonstrating that not only did class inequalities still exist but they were getting worse and also there were inequalities associated with race and gender, which had yet to be articulated.

Inequality since the 1990s

Inequality remained in the wings of the NHS policy-making stage in the 1980s but in the 1990s the climate changed. The WHO's regional strategy for Europe (WHO 1985) and the *Health of the Nation* (Department of Health 1992) to which it gave rise (see Chapter 9) contributed to a greater willingness to accept the notion of class differences in health and the need to tackle these if overall health is to be improved. Thus, some of Black's recommendations were taken on board through the *Health of the Nation* targets. These tended to be directed at those conditions characterized by class gradients such as coronary heart disease, strokes and lung cancer and the behaviours associated with them such as smoking and alcohol consumption.

The need to address unequal access to health services is acknowledged in the system of paying GPs, which is so arranged that extra fees are payable for patients living in deprived areas. There are many creative outreach and other programmes designed to improve access for poorer citizens, and this is an aspect of health care provision which PCTs and HAs are now called upon to address via Investment Plans and Health Improvement Programmes (HImPs). But inequality in health and health care has continued to prove intractable. Indeed, the gulf between those at the top of the social ladder and those at the bottom is growing (Graham 1997; Mitchell *et al.* 2000; Office of National Statistics 1997; Wilkinson 1996). There is a marked differential between the mortality rates of men in social classes I–IV whose death rates have steadily declined since the 1970s and those of men in social class V for whom death rates were higher in 1992–93 than they had been twenty years earlier (see Table 7.1).

Table 7.1 Male standardized mortality ratios by social class, 1920s–90s

Decade	I	II	III	IV	V
1920s	88	95	96	100	125
1930s	90	92	96	100	108
1950s	82	90	100	105	120
1960s	72	80	98	102	140
1970s	72	80	100	113	138
1980s	63	72	95	113	160
1990s	63	68	100	118	188

Source: based on Graham (1997, p. 15)

In 1997, a five-year, inter-disciplinary project exploring the causes of variations in health was launched, funded by the Economic and Social Research Council.

Explaining inequality

The health inequality debate revolves around two contrasting positions. First is the 'conservative' view, which sees health as the responsibility of the individual and illness as a problem that can be solved without changing the class structure. The health of the poor can be improved by persuading them to copy the lifestyle of the healthier middle classes. Such a stance may allow that poverty plays a part in ill health but only *in extremis*. As long as there is *sufficient* income, with sensible budgeting and access to the NHS, a healthy lifestyle can be attained. This position is difficult to sustain, however, in view of the widening inequalities in the UK over the past fifty years (see Table 7.1) despite a universal NHS and huge rises in the standard of living.

By contrast, the 'radical environmentalists' place more emphasis on structural factors than behaviour as contributors to ill health and recognize that the complex relationship between health and poverty can be understood only in terms of social class, of which occupation is an important part.

Occupation affects health in very direct ways. Certain jobs expose their members to high risk of illness or injury. Some job-related illnesses have long been recognized, like the 'phossy jaw' to which girls working in match factories were subject in the nineteenth century; the scrotal cancer which claimed the lives of many young chimney sweeps; and the respiratory conditions which long afflicted miners. Although much has been done to make work safer, the link between occupation and health remains. The high rate of cervical cancer among working-class women may, for example, be due to their contact with harmful chemicals inadvertently brought home by husbands who work in dusty jobs. Furthermore, there is greater awareness of the less direct ill-effects of higher levels of job insecurity and low pay.

Occupation also largely determines income. Income is the single most important factor in housing, environment and diet, all of which have a direct effect on health. Poor housing contributes to respiratory illness, inner city living is likely to trigger and aggravate asthma and the poor are less likely to be in a position to afford a healthy diet.

It should not, therefore, be assumed that the poor have chosen their lifestyle and that health promotion depends on persuading them to change. In areas where there is choice, the effects of poverty may be such that healthy choices are not the most

attractive. Where behaviour does have an effect, it is more pro-
nounced among those whose socio-economic environment is good,
i.e. healthy behaviour reinforces advantage to a much greater extent
than unhealthy behaviour reinforces disadvantage. (For further discussion of lifestyle and choice, see Chapter 10.)

It is difficult to disentangle the effects of social class from those
of lifestyle. In carrying out a health audit, Wakefield HA made no
such attempt. It recognized the influence of both its long history of
mining and high levels of smoking in contributing to higher than
average rates of heart disease and cancers (Wakefield Health
Authority 1997).

One device that offers a way of tackling class-based inequalities
is social indicators. These are characteristics known to be associated
with deprivation such as the number of single parent families or the
level of unemployment. These can be used to identify inequalities
and to target efforts to improve access to health care for disadvantaged groups. For example, the Jarman underprivileged area score
was used in the health audit undertaken by Wakefield HA
(Wakefield Health Authority 1997) and could be used to inform
resource allocation decisions more generally.

The international perspective

Interest in health inequalities has extended beyond national boundaries and research shows that, internationally, the link between
poverty and ill health is not straightforward. 'Life expectancy is
[generally] higher in countries like Greece, Japan, Iceland and Italy
than it is in richer countries like the United States or Germany'
(Wilkinson 1996, p. 2). When a society reaches a stage of economic
development such that adequate material living standards can be
provided for everyone, further growth does not continue to generate overall improvements in health.

Arrival at this stage is marked by the 'epidemiological transition', that is, the point at which infectious diseases give way to
cancers and degenerative conditions as the major causes of death.
Moreover, these diseases, once considered the diseases of affluence,
become the diseases of the poor in affluent societies.

The key to health appears to lie not in the total amount of wealth but rather in the manner in which it is distributed, with those societies displaying the most equal distribution having the best standard of health. 'It is now clear that the scale of income differences in a society is one of the most powerful determinants of health standards in different countries' (Wilkinson 1996, p. ix). We now know 'it is not the richest countries which have the best health but the most egalitarian' (ibid., p. 3).

A possible explanation for this is that income inequality undermines social cohesion, thereby harming the social fabric and damaging health (ibid.). The health of everyone living in an unequal society suffers, not simply those who are least well off. The equality argument has, in a sense, come back to the Black Report.

Class and employment

Not only do the poor experience worse health and inferior access to health services, but their opportunities for employment in the NHS are limited by their position in the social structure. The NHS is a microcosm of the wider social system, with a class structure similar to that of the society it serves.

At the top are the mainly London-based consultants who are able to combine NHS practice with lucrative private work. Around 500 consultants earn over £150,000 per year with the highest incomes going to those in fields such as plastic surgery, dermatology and gynaecology. Merit awards (received by approximately one-third of consultants) mean that some 250 consultants earn more than £100,000 a year from the NHS alone (Adonis and Pollard 1997). The privileged position of consultants is part of a long-standing, unwritten and barely acknowledged agreement with the medical profession, which serves to keep the medical elite within the NHS, rather than encouraging them to succumb to the lure of the private sector.

The next level in the hierarchy is the upper-middle class, comprising the less well off consultants and senior managers. A typical NHS Trust chief executive receives around £70,000 a year. The middle class, GPs on an average in excess of £50,000 a year, and hospital registrars, are still better remunerated than the middle class in general. Then comes the skilled, lower-middle class of mainly female nurses, therapists, technologists and technicians earning in the region of £13,000 a year. Finally, the medical proletariat at the bottom includes auxiliary, ancillary and service staff. Apart from hospital porters, this group is overwhelmingly female. Their pay has remained at a constant level for the last decade (£6,000 a year for cleaners), while the salaries of top managers have soared (Adonis and Pollard 1997).

Gender

Women as users

Women make greater use of health services than men for a number of reasons. Maternity and gynaecological services are used exclusively by women and their longer life expectancy also contributes to their disproportionate use of services. Additionally, their position in the family means that they are more likely to take the major responsibility for the health of family members, acting as a conduit between them and formal services, and determining diet, lifestyle and many aspects of the physical environment.

However, they also appear to make greater use of services on their own behalf (Smith 1987; Reid and Stratta 1989; Research Unit in Health and Behavioural Change 1989). A complex interplay of social and biological factors underlie this situation including how health is defined and viewed by women and professionals and the self-image of women.

Yet all too often the NHS has not been mindful of the needs of women. At a very practical level, the location and timing of clinics, hospital visiting times, the design of buildings and the availability of facilities for children have made it difficult for women, particularly if they are employed outside the home and do not have access to private transport. The cultural gap between clinicians and many of their female patients has sometimes meant that advice and services are given in a way which displays a lack of understanding, sensitivity and realism with respect to the everyday lives of patients.

More profoundly, since the mid-1970s, health care has become of increasing concern to feminists who have criticized its patriarchal nature. A particular concern is the medicalization of reproduction, which has led to the control of women's reproductive lives by (predominantly) male professionals. Feminist writers point to the fact that women's access to fertility treatments, contraception and abortion, decisions about where and how to give birth and how to manage the menopause are mediated by a patriarchal medical profession. (See Dale and Foster 1986; Williams 1989; Foster 1995; Pascall 1996; Annandale and Hunt 1999.)

Medical and scientific knowledge in these matters is not incontrovertible, but is informed by prevailing values and beliefs. Because these are deeply embedded, the knowledge is not questioned nor are the decisions to which it gives rise; they become the orthodoxy. We come to believe that childbirth is dangerous and should take place in hospital; postnatal depression is a hormonal imbalance; and the menopause is a treatable, hormone deficiency disease. Women are often, therefore, not told about alternative treatments and are not invited to contribute to their own health care.

The Women's Health Movement

It was not until the 1960s that there was any real insight into these issues or systematic attempts to suggest alternatives. Such attempts, when they did come, can be summed up as the Women's Health Movement. Although something of a muddle of loosely related groups and approaches, the movement is unified in its challenge to the patriarchal culture of modern medicine and to conventional medical therapies. Its principles are those of:

- greater sharing of knowledge and control
- blurring the distinction between professionals and patients
- flatter hierarchies.

Four general approaches are associated with the Women's Health Movement. First, imported from the USA, is collective action such as local women's health groups where women learn about their bodies as a first step to taking control of their health. Second, is the concept of the women's health centre where, to a greater or lesser extent, the principles of non-patriarchal health care are put into practice. The third approach is based on self-help groups which can cover a range of conditions affecting women such as pre-menstrual tension, eating disorders, cystitis and postnatal depression. Finally, there is political action such as Action for Improvement in Maternity Services and the Campaign for Natural Childbirth. Interestingly, in parallel with the feminist challenge to the patriarchy endemic in the NHS, there has been a much more broadly based disaffection with modern medical care (see Chapter 9), which has served to legitimize the Women's Health Movement and give its strategies wider applicability. A primary care-led NHS in which community-based health promotion and illness prevention and low-tech, simple treatments move centre stage is compatible with the aims and practice of the Women's Health Movement.

Women in health care

As well as being major users of health care, women also play a key role as formal and informal providers (see Chapter 3). In the past women were the healers; they cared for the sick and dying, assisted one another in childbirth and had elaborate and well-developed remedies for simple ailments, many of which were subsequently 'proved' to be effective (Ehrenreich and English 1973; Versluyen 1980; Towler and Bramall 1986). Indeed, health care was considered 'women's work', too menial and dirty to be of interest to men.

However, from the end of the seventeenth century, through the twin processes of technocratization and professionalization, men gradually colonized health work. Women healers were dismissed as amateurish, ill informed and dangerous (an image immortalized in Charles Dickens' character, Sarah Gamp). Men brought science into the business of health, thereby removing it from the informal, lay arena and placing it firmly in the exclusive professional domain. Health care providers had to be formally trained in scientific skills and, since men dominated education, they were able to exclude women and outrun them in career advancement. For example, in the field of midwifery, the invention of forceps, which women were not trained to use, effectively paved the way for the development of the separate and gendered career paths of obstetrics and midwifery.

The health care role was not lost to women but it was redefined in the context of a male-dominated medical profession. And, since much of this process took place in the nineteenth century, it is hardly surprising that the professional roles that emerged for men and women were consistent with prevailing Victorian norms. Women were the nurses and men the doctors; women the carers and men the curers. The role of the nurse simply did not exist until the doctor had diagnosed the condition and prescribed a course of treatment, which it then became the nurse's responsibility to administer.

Although women did break into medicine in the closing years of the nineteenth century, it was not until the latter half of the twentieth century that they seriously began to challenge its patriarchal nature and fight to reclaim their lost territory. The development of the concept of the nursing process and the changes to nurse education embodied in Project 2000 symbolized the desire to re-establish nursing as an autonomous profession. Campaigns such as that to promote natural childbirth and the altercations between Wendy Savage and her male obstetric colleagues in 1986 similarly bear witness to a radical attempt to recover ground lost by women healers and their patients.

Table 7.2 Hospital medical staff, 2000

Grade	Total*	Male (%)	Female (%)
Total	57,940.9	67	33
Consultant	21,076.5	79	21
Staff Grade	3,763.7	69	31
Associate Specialist	1,332.7	69	31
Registrar Group	11,675.9	64	36
Senior House Officer	14,886.8	55	45
House Officer	3,634.2	50	50
Hospital Practitioner	183.3	77	23
Clinical Assistant	1,386.8	58	42

* Whole time equivalents
Source: Department of Health (2000a)

Table 7.3 Community dental staff, 2000

Grade	Total*	Male (%)	Female (%)
Total	997.1	38	62
Clinical Director	60.2	54	46
Senior Dental Officer	338.6	42	58
Dental Officer	469.2	28	72

* Whole time equivalents
Source: Department of Health (2000a)

Table 7.4 NHS hospital and community health services nursing, midwifery and health visiting staff by sex, 2000

Grade	Total	Male (%)	Female (%)
Total	346,176	13	87
Managers	4,579	22	78

Source: Department of Health (2000a)

Table 7.5 Public health medicine (PHM) and community health service medical staff, 2000

Grade	Total*	Male (%)	Female (%)
Total	1,728.3	43	57
District Director of Public Health	93.9	61	39
Consultant in PHM	500.3	57	43
Senior Registrar in PHM	49.1	35	65
Senior House Officer in PHM	31.2	33	67
Senior Clinical Medical Officer	465.4	35	65
Clinical Medical Officer	293.8	24	76

* Whole time equivalents
Source: Department of Health (2000a)

Women and the NHS

Today the NHS remains a popular occupational choice for women, with over 80 per cent of NHS employees being female (Department of Health 2000a). But they are over-represented in low-tech, practical jobs that involve the most patient contact and are more to do with caring than curing. They are also over-represented at the lower levels of the organizational hierarchy (see Tables 7.2–7.5).

There are numerous explanations for this state of affairs:

- Women are seen and see themselves as less suitable for or interested in high level jobs.
- Potential role conflict for women seeking to combine a career with a domestic role may make them reluctant to put themselves forward and employers reluctant to select them, particularly as working arrangements tend to become less flexible at higher levels.
- The culture of the NHS at senior levels is still white, male and middle class. This likely to be viewed as an inhospitable climate by women themselves and it is also likely to perpetuate itself.

The pertinence of the domestic role for working women was highlighted in a study carried out by the NHS Women's Unit in 1994 of the career paths of NHS managers. It found that, among top managers:

- 23 per cent of women were single compared with 2 per cent of men
- 7 per cent of women had children compared with 90 per cent of men
- women devoted forty-three hours to domestic duties compared with the seventeen hours undertaken by men (NHS Women's Unit 1994).

In short, there is a potent amalgam of institutional, ideological and behavioural discrimination.

Impact of discrimination against women

Although it would be quite wrong to pursue this line of argument too far, it is probably fair to say that gender divisions within NHS work have moulded its culture and practices. For example, the slow development of primary care teams and the wrangles over leadership of such teams, discussed in Chapter 9, suggest that the NHS tends towards hierarchies and authoritarian structures rather than teamwork. Arguably, this reflects the patriarchal culture since teamwork may be a more natural way of working for women than men. The culture of the NHS also reflects the dominance of men in the sense that certain types of health care – those low-tech, preventive services located in the community where women tend to predominate, have generally been less highly regarded and rewarded than the more scientifically based, high-tech hospital services for which male professionals show a preference.

Race

Inequalities associated with race have been recognized only relatively recently and the evidence is therefore sparse (Law 1996). This is due mainly to the absence of ethnic monitoring; it was not until the 1991 census, for example, that official statistics included race. There is now, however, a growing body of research which suggests that people from minority ethnic groups living in poverty experience worse health than other groups in Britain (see Nazroo 1997; Karlsen and Nazroo 2000).

Members of minority ethnic communities are over-represented in the lower socio-economic groups and are, therefore, likely to experience poverty and hence poor housing, schools, diet and environment. To some extent, therefore, their health status is a function of their socio-economic status, and it is mistaken to interpret too much as a result of race when the problem is one of class. However, it is difficult to disentangle the effects of class and race.

The health of minority ethnic groups

Some conditions are unusual or non-existent among the white population. The best known examples are sickle cell disease (mainly affecting Afro-Caribbeans); rickets (mainly affecting Asians); and the health problems caused by the long-acting contraceptive

Depoprovera, disproportionately prescribed to black women. Afro-Caribbeans have a greater chance of being diagnosed as suffering from one of the more serious forms of mental illness, including schizophrenia, which may reflect real differences but is more likely to be the outcome of prejudice or the expectations of professionals. Asians are particularly vulnerable to heart disease and diabetes. Black and Asian women are more likely to suffer from cervical cancer. However, in other respects the effects of race are less easy to identify and the health profile of minority ethnic communities looks very similar to that of the lower social classes in general, e.g. they display a higher than average incidence of anaemias and tuberculosis (which is linked to homelessness).

Similarly, indicators of health behaviour suggest a strong resemblance between members of minority ethnic groups and the working classes generally. For example, mothers born in the countries of the New Commonwealth have low take up of antenatal and postnatal services; they are more likely to have low birth-weight babies and a higher infant mortality rate; and they are less likely to make the link between weight and health (Skellington 1996).

Race and health care

The evidence suggests that the NHS generally provides poorer care for minority ethnic groups. Cumberlege is unequivocal on this matter, 'We are finding that people with minority ethnic backgrounds do not get the full benefit of NHS services and this applies at all levels: access . . . treatment and outcome' (Cumberlege, in Skellington 1996, p. 120). Mohammed says that the response of the NHS 'has in all but a few cases been either to neglect or to marginalize the needs of their black populations' (Mohammed, in Skellington 1996, pp. 119–120).

Members of minority ethnic communities not only wait longer for treatment (for heart disease, for example) and receive poorer quality coronary care; they also do less well in the field of health promotion. This was highlighted by two surveys carried out in 1995 by the Health Education Authority and the King's Fund. Significant numbers of respondents had not received any health information; there was a lack of interest in information about alcohol, drug abuse and contraception; nearly a third of Indian women and nearly a half of Pakistani women had never been screened for cervical cancer; and a third of Indian men who smoked did not know of the likely effects of smoking on health (Health Education Authority and the King's Fund 1995 a, b).

Here again, it is difficult to unravel class and race. There are cultural barriers that prevent members of minority ethnic groups from making the best use of health care services. Language differences impede both written and spoken communication. There may also be problems of unfamiliarity with complex organizations, feeling ill at ease with professional service providers, the absence of a female doctor if required, an appropriate diet in hospitals and procedures that demonstrate respect for religious beliefs and cultural norms. All these can serve to flaw encounters with health care services and may even deter members of minority ethnic groups from using services. Cultural diversity demands diverse services, yet the NHS has demonstrably failed to overcome cultural barriers and provide a service that is genuinely accessible to everyone. It has instead been concerned with establishing uniform practices and standardized services – paradoxically in the interests of securing equal health services for all – but this will inevitably be unacceptable to those who do not share the dominant cultural values. 'It is clear that the . . . services . . . have been slow to accommodate to the changing needs of an increasing multi-ethnic and multicultural society' (Johnson, in Skellington 1996, p. 112). In principle, these are issues that could be tackled through informed and sensitive service planning and delivery. More profound, however, are racist ideologies and the racial harassment to which they give rise (Law 1996, p. 149).

Righting the wrongs

A number of official circulars and publications throughout the 1970s and 1980s appeared to have little impact (Law 1996). But in 1991, a press release from the Department of Health seemed to usher in a more determined disposition. It stated that 'Health Authorities are expected to provide services that are acceptable to members of minority ethnic communities. This involves positive action to take account of differences in language, culture and religion' (Department of Health 1991c). Two years later, the message was stronger, stressing the importance of sensitivity to the needs of minority ethnic groups and genuine equity of access and provision.

True to the spirit of these statements, in 1993 the NHS Executive established, for a period of three years, the NHS Ethnic Health Unit to encourage purchasers and providers to improve access for minority ethnic groups. Its purpose was to help HAs and NHS Trusts ensure that minority ethnic people derive full benefit from the NHS. It sought, amongst other things, to ensure that minority ethnic groups had a say in decisions on purchasing and service provision and to fund initiatives designed to promote partnerships between purchasers and providers and local minority ethnic groups. The Unit was disbanded, as planned, in 1996 in the belief that it had achieved some degree of awareness raising, but judgements of its efficacy are mixed.

Also in 1993, the Commission for Racial Equality (CRE) launched the Race Relations Code of Practice in Primary Health Care Services. The document was designed to elaborate on legislation by giving guidelines regarding implementation and good practice. However, as its status fell short of that of legislation, little notice was taken of it (Law 1996).

Many commentators stress the importance of ensuring that those who design services and determine their mode of delivery should be representative of service users or, at least, solicit the views of all service users. Abercrombie and Warde (1995) argue that measures to rectify the position of minority ethnic groups have had little impact partly due to the fact that the ethnic minorities themselves have had little involvement. In 1993, the Secretary of State launched an eight-point plan to secure equitable representation of minority ethnic groups at all levels in the NHS. Clearly such a strategy will take time to have an effect and it is too soon to judge its impact.

Race and employment

The NHS is the largest employer of minority ethnic people in Britain, this group constituting 9 per cent of the workforce (Law

1996; Jack 1999). By 1975, 20.5 per cent of all student and pupil nurses in Britain were from overseas and about half of them had been recruited in their country of origin (Jones 1994), and this continues to be a contentious issue.

However, despite their substantial numbers, members of minority ethnic groups are not adequately represented at senior levels (see Table 7.6), and consequently have a weak voice in the policy-making arena. They are concentrated in the least prestigious and lowest grades of medicine and nursing. For example, members of minority ethnic groups are more frequently found among enrolled, pupil and auxiliary nurses partly because the education requirements are less, but also because the entry qualifications for State Registered Nurse are geared to British educational criteria (Jones 1994). They are over-represented in the less popular and prestigious medical specialisms such as geriatrics and psychiatry and in ancillary posts such as domestic, catering, cleaning and maintenance. In general, members of minority ethnic groups have less training, their promotion prospects are poorer and salaries are lower.

Table 7.6 Hospital medical staff by ethnic origin and grade, 2000 (%)

Grade	White	Black	Asian	Other
All staff	64	5	20	9
Consultant	79	3	10	7
Staff Grade	32	10	38	19
Associate Specialist	33	7	35	23
Registrar Group	63	5	23	8
Senior House Officer	56	5	28	9
House Officer	63	4	20	8
Hospital Practitioner	79	1	12	5
Clinical Assistant	61	4	23	11

Source: Department of Health (2000a)

Whereas the dual role of women helps to explain their poorer prospects, there is no equivalent rationale for minority ethnic groups. There is, however, evidence of the part played by discrimination in determining employment opportunities: from the institutional racism of rules and regulations that work to their disadvantage down to the racism of fellow workers. In 1988, the CRE formally investigated St George's Hospital Medical School and found evidence of direct discrimination on racial grounds contrary to the Race Relations Act 1976. Interestingly, the discrimination occurred through the operation of the school's computerized admissions and selection procedure; the system was discriminatory although the institution itself was liberal (Skellington 1996).

Evidence of discrimination has also been gathered by researchers making a series of bogus applications to the NHS. Two applications were submitted for a number of advertised posts. The applications were identical in every respect but the name: one being Anglo-Saxon and the other Asian. In every case the former candidate was much more likely to be called for interview than the latter (Bagilhole 1997).

The disadvantaged position of members of minority ethnic groups in the NHS clearly has implications for the individuals themselves: their career development, standard of living, status, self-esteem and so forth. But it also has implications for the design and delivery of health services. Health services will continue to bear the stamp of the white, European, male culture as long as such individuals dominate decision-making. With mounting recruitment problems, the increasingly multi-cultural nature of our society and the challenge of providing a health service that is accessible and acceptable to all citizens, such a culture is perhaps too narrow. Indeed, the Race Relations (Amendment) Act 2000 prohibits any public organization from discriminating on grounds of race in carrying out its functions; in the case of the NHS this covers both its employment policies and the services it provides.

Equal opportunities in the NHS

More assertive feminist and anti-racist movements in society at large set the scene for an equal opportunities agenda within the NHS in the last quarter of the twentieth century. Like many other organizations, the NHS has been called upon to devise policies and codes of practice to promote equality of opportunity and to protect the interests of minority groups in employment. By the 1990s, most parts of the NHS had such policies in place but few 'had translated [policies] into a timetabled programme for action or had allocated responsibilities or resources' (Equal Opportunities Task Force, in Skellington 1996, p. 119). By 2001 only 5 per cent of NHS Trusts had fully implemented equality programmes and the CRE expressed disappointment that the NHS workforce did not reflect Britain's multi-racial society (Commission for Racial Equality 2001).

Nevertheless, the existence of a formal statement is important. It helps to raise and maintain awareness of equal opportunity issues, it gives pause for thought with respect to the employment needs of minority groups and can be used by those committed to change. Certainly, in recent years, more systematic attention has been given to a number of matters relating to both the physical work environment and to employment procedures and practices. For example:

- the provision of workplace nurseries and prayer rooms for Muslims
- ensuring that recruitment, training, staff development and promotion procedures are systematic, visible and fair
- giving equal pay for work of equal value
- making working practices acceptable in terms of hours of work and flexibility
- introducing flexible contracts and career breaks
- securing a workplace culture of mutual respect and support, which genuinely welcomes diversity.

A somewhat controversial approach to equal opportunities is positive action, defined as any measure intended to redress the effects of previous unequal practice. The most visible example of this is Opportunity 2000, a campaign to increase the quantity and quality of women's participation in the workforce. The Department of Health committed the NHS to investing in management and personal development targeted at women in more junior levels and women from minority ethnic groups. The campaign produced:

- targeted advertising
- training programmes
- shadowing schemes
- surveys of women's views
- equal opportunities targets in staff appraisal at all levels
- steps to increase the number of women returning after maternity leave
- monitoring mechanisms.

The Programme of Action for Ethnic Minority Staff in the NHS is another example of positive action. In 1994–95, £250,000 was set aside for management development for minority ethnic staff and for attracting members of minority ethnic groups into speech therapy.

Target setting is another strategy associated with equal opportunities, but also subject to controversy. Clearly, it is good practice to monitor the effects of equal opportunities programmes, and targets relating to the number of women or black people employed in various parts of the NHS is a device for this purpose. Moreover, the proponents of targets argue that, since the purpose of equal opportunities initiatives is to increase the numbers of employees from minority groups at various levels in the hierarchy, we must be prepared to quantify this objective and measure progress.

Critics of target-setting argue, however, that it is difficult to know where to set the targets. If they are too high, they are unrealistic and defeatism may set in. If they are too low, complacency may result. Target-setting can lead to an undue emphasis on quantifiable issues at the expense of equally important, non-quantifiable matters. The targets may not be sufficiently flexible to reflect the different circumstances and requirements of different parts of the organization.

In its commitment to Opportunity 2000, the NHS set a number of targets relating to women's employment. For example, between 1991 and 1994 there was to be an increase of:

- women in general management posts from 18 to 30 per cent
- qualified female accountants to 35 per cent
- women consultants from 15.5 to 20 per cent.

In the event, by 1994 38 per cent of general managers, 31 per cent of accountants and 17 per cent of consultants were women (by 2001 the percentage of women consultants had risen to 21 – see Table 7.2).

Looking to the future

Inequalities in health, health care and employment in the NHS have been persistent. At their heart lies lack of power, rooted deep in the structure of society and mediated by the political and economic environment.

Trends in the wider society since the early 1990s may have made it harder to tackle inequalities. Growing levels of income inequality and the larger role for the 'macho' commercial sector sit uneasily with equality measures. Moreover, Trusts have been preoccupied with financial and organizational issues and anything regarded as peripheral, such as equality initiatives, is likely to be seen as dispensable. It is also possible that, despite continued research and growing understanding of the issues, the 'hard edge' has gone off anti-discrimination movements.

Against this has to be set a number of wider trends which both necessitate and legitimize equality. Demographic trends are changing the composition of the workforce; epidemiological and technological changes are transforming the nature and cost of health care. The influence of Europe is restricting the freedom of choice of decision-makers within the NHS. In other words, Britain may have equality thrust upon it. More generally, there is some evidence that the 'macho' culture of the 1980s and 1990s is giving way to a softer climate, in which fairness and justice are given a higher priority than has been the custom in the recent past.

Key points

- Despite wide acceptance of the principle of equal access to health care and equality of opportunity in employment, it is apparent that certain groups have done less well than others in the health care system.

- Growing awareness of the health needs of the poor, women and members of minority ethnic groups and more sophisticated understanding of the mechanisms of discrimination have done much to publicize the issues and, undoubtedly, some improvements have been achieved.

- There are powerful moral, legal and socio-economic arguments for equalizing opportunities.

- Social class inequalities in health and health care were brought to the fore by the Black Report but since then little has improved and, in some respects, things have deteriorated. Continued research has contributed to a growing understanding of class inequalities in health, health care and employment in the NHS, and their relationship with the structure of the wider society.

- Women use health services more than men, yet there is evidence that services are neither designed nor delivered in a way that meets their needs. This critique gave rise to the Women's Health Movement, but it has had only a limited impact on mainstream health services.

- Women have a traditional role as providers of health care and continue to play a large part in the NHS but predominantly in the low-tech, practical, caring roles at the lower levels of the hierarchy. This can be explained in terms of both their dual role and discrimination and it has, undoubtedly, had an impact on the culture and practice of the NHS.

- The poorer health and health care experienced by members of minority ethnic groups is related both to socio-economic status and to discrimination. Recent measures to tackle these problems have had a limited effect.

- As employees, members of minority ethnic groups are over-represented at the lower levels of the NHS and in the least prestigious branches of the professions. This is explained in terms of discrimination.

- Like most large organizations, the NHS has put in place a range of Equal Opportunities initiatives but wrestles with the vexed questions of how to monitor their impact and ensure their effectiveness.

Guide to further reading

M. Powell's (1997) *Evaluating the National Health Service*, Buckingham: Open University Press, gives good coverage of inequalities associated with class, race and gender in the context of evaluating the NHS.

For an international perspective on health inequalities, R.C. Wilkinson's (1996) *Unhealthy Societies: The Afflictions of Inequality*, London: Routledge, is essential reading. The book is based on research linking the health status of populations with the degree of income inequality.

L. Jones's (1994) *The Social Context of Health and Health Work*, London: Macmillan, provides useful further reading on this subject. In Chapter 5 she looks at class-based inequalities in health; in Chapter 6 the health effects of poverty; in Chapter 7 gender and health status; and in Chapter 8 the health and health care experiences of minority ethnic groups. The debate is conducted in the context of sociological theories of class, gender and race and debates about race and ethnicity.

Chapter 10 of R. Baggott's (2000) *Public Health: Policy and Politics*, Basingstoke: Macmillan, is a useful overview.

An accessible introduction to the key arguments, problems and research findings in the field of women's health is provided by A. Miles (1991) in *Women, Health and Medicine*, Buckingham: Open University Press.

A useful introduction to the whole area of equal opportunities, particularly for students of social policy, is B. Bagilhole (1997) *Equal Opportunities and Social Policy*, London: Longman. The book also includes a chapter dedicated to health and housing services.

Although concentrating on the private sector, R. Kandola and J. Fullerton (1994) *Managing the Mosaic: Diversity in Action*, London: Institute of Personnel and Development, present a convincing case for equal opportunities in employment which is as applicable to the NHS as to the organizations that are the focus of this book.

A. Adonis and S. Pollard's (1997) *Class Act: Myth of Britain's Classless Society*, London: Hamilton (Hamish) Ltd., offers a lively and provocative analysis of class divisions in employment in the NHS.

I. Law's (1996) *Racism, Ethnicity and Social Policy*, London: Prentice-Hall/Harvester Wheatsheaf, contains an excellent chapter on 'Ethnicity and Health: Problems and Policies'.

Part III

The future – new possibilities

Chapter 8
The mixed economy of health

OUTLINE
Pressure on the NHS and ideological shifts in the last quarter of the twentieth century raised the profile of both the voluntary and commercial sectors of health care. The health care pluralist argument is that the source of health care is relatively unimportant, so long as the care is provided. An examination of each sector – their characteristics, constraints and shortcomings – suggests that they are not interchangeable, however, and any shift in the balance between them should be carefully considered. Furthermore, each sector has undergone profound recent change, making the distinction between them less clear.

Introduction

Health care has always been provided by a variety of agents, including those in the informal, voluntary and commercial sectors, as well as the NHS. The balance between the sectors has been an ever moving picture and the distinction between them increasingly less sharp. Chapter 3 looked at these various sectors, their history and the manner in which their role developed in the postwar years. Chapter 6 examined the impact of managerialism on culture, ownership, control and access in the NHS. This chapter will consider the future in the light of both past developments and recent trends.

It is likely that, in the future, health care will come from a greater variety of sources than has recently been the case. Growing doubts about the NHS's ability to meet contemporary challenges, together with governments' reduction of the size and influence of the public sector since 1979, have already produced a radical restructuring of welfare and a strategic shift away from the NHS. This may be interpreted as healthy diversity or as fragmentation of the health care system. In examining each of these views, the terms 'welfare pluralism' or 'mixed economy of health' have been used (Mishra 1990).

The mixed economy of health

The sectors involved in the delivery of health care can be defined by two criteria, namely, ownership (that is, whether the resources are owned publicly or privately) and principles governing eligibility (that is, whether access to such resources is on the basis of the individual's ability and willingness to pay, or need). Table 8.1 illustrates the distinction.

Table 8.1 Ownership and eligibility

Eligibility	Public ownership	Private ownership
On basis of ability and willingness to pay	Nationalized industries	Commercial organizations, e.g. private hospitals
On basis of need	NHS	Voluntary

Because of the dominance of the NHS since 1948, and the clear dividing lines between the NHS and the other sectors, the involvement of the different sectors has tended to be obscured. This is no longer the case. Demarcation lines are less clear; multi-sectoral involvement has a much higher profile and the important part played by sectors other than the NHS cannot be overlooked.

The health care pluralist debate

The welfare pluralist argument states that:

> welfare derives from a multitude of sources: the State, the market (including enterprise), voluntary and charitable organizations and the kinship network (including household). To equate social welfare with State welfare is therefore to ignore all of these other sources of social protection and support.

Total welfare in a society is a sum of these parts. The diminution of one of the welfare sectors does not necessarily mean a net loss of welfare.

(Mishra 1990, p. 108)

It follows that recent changes in health care can be seen simply as a shift of emphasis from one sector to another.

Welfare pluralists argue that 'a crisis of the Welfare State is not a crisis of welfare in society' (Rose, in Mishra 1990, p. 110) and they point to successful examples of welfare pluralism such as the Netherlands. The argument that one sector will automatically compensate for another, however, is unsound. While there is evidence to suggest that the State takes over when the informal and commercial sectors are struggling (district nursing and health visiting in the early years of the twentieth century and hospitals in the 1940s), there is only partial evidence to suggest that if the State gets into difficulties or wishes to withdraw, the other two sectors will step up their pace.

Furthermore, although the tasks of providing health care may be very similar, whether they are carried out in the public, commercial or voluntary sector, the goals and context will be quite distinct (Ranson and Stewart 1994), which means they are not equally suitable in all circumstances. The future of health care should be informed by an understanding of the different contributions that the sectors can and should make.

Public service

Rationale

In 1948, traditional health care markets were rejected in favour of a tax-funded public service, which allocated resources according to need (see Table 8.1). 'The reasons for providing a service in the first place, the nature of that service and the manner in which it is delivered, are not dictated by markets but by needs and the availability of resources' (Lawton and Rose 1994, p. 7). Arguably, health care is too important to be left to the vagaries of the market. It confers external benefits, that is the benefit of any health care intervention is experienced not only by the individual receiving it but also by society at large. In other words, in providing health care, the government is pursuing social goals that profit-seeking, market-oriented, private sector organizations overlook or play down. These social goals may be said to include:

- stability – avoiding inequality along health lines and the consequent resentment this engenders, removing anxiety associated with health costs
- efficiency – contributing to the good health of the next generation of employees, ensuring that ill health does not undermine the ability of people to fill their social roles as parents and citizens
- safety – protecting people from disease and the fear of disease, minimizing the potential for epidemics.

The NHS, therefore, embodies governments' cumulative decisions to distribute health resources according to social principles. The NHS pursues collective values expressed through collective choice and serves citizens, not just customers. In this way, individual health is promoted, not as an end in itself, but as the means to a stable, efficient and safe society. There is a danger, however, that over time, this end becomes obscured and the promotion of individual health comes to be seen as the major element. Hence, the NHS acquires a strong moral component, to be either defended as the mark of a civilized society or attacked as compounding the 'nanny State'. The former argument rests on the notion that health is a social right of citizenship, and should neither depend on the individual's ability to pay nor generate profit for those with the power to bestow it. The latter argument is justified on the grounds that freedom of choice is part of being a mature human being and that the NHS removes the need to choose.

Nature of public service

As a public service, the NHS has certain characteristics:

- Its objectives are multiple, vague and ill-defined, focusing both on the individual and society. This makes the formulation and implementation of policy highly complex, and the evaluation of performance and outcomes difficult and contestable.

- Because funds are raised through taxation, spending is related to overall economic performance.
- The NHS operates in a highly politicized context. Spending is likely to depend as much on political factors as economic ones. Policy is largely determined by politicians and is, therefore, subject to short termism.
- Public accountability means that the NHS operates under the public gaze. Its broadly democratic setting is elaborated, because of perceived inadequacies in representative government, by a number of alternative forms of representation such as the Health Service Ombudsman, CHCs and patient forums.
- The service itself has been organized as a bureaucracy. Protected from the competitive world of the market, bureaucrats have little incentive to reduce costs or operate efficiently but strong incentives to fight to increase their share of resources.
- The NHS has many different stakeholders (consumers, patients, taxpayers, citizens, politicians and the media). Thus, an important part of managing the health service is balancing competing interests (Lawton and Rose 1994) (see Chapter 5).
- For those working in the NHS, there is 'a public service ethic which was part of the post-war consensus and emphasizes collective responsibility for certain services, equitable treatment of people regardless of their incomes, and includes a belief that it is wrong to make profits from essential services' (Flynn 1993, p. 184).

Perhaps this is an outmoded stereotype. Since the early 1980s the NHS has been radically reshaped in a way sometimes described as 'creeping privatization', 'marketization' and 'radicalism by stealth' (Baggott 1998). Service providers have been obliged to adopt the enterprise culture, including business-style management, commercial values and market mechanisms. As a result, the NHS much less resembles the stereotypical public sector organization of earlier decades (see Chapter 6). Nevertheless, these characteristics give a sense of what the public sector is about, how it is constrained and the challenges it is likely to face if it continues to be a major provider of health care in Britain.

The voluntary sector

The voluntary sector has a much longer history than the public sector. It was the only source of support for those in need before public services emerged, thus trail-blazing modern health services for the government. Since then it has stood the test of time, surviving:

- the heyday of the Welfare State
- the changing role of women in society
- changing family patterns
- community care policies
- the epidemiological transition
- the ageing of the population.

This longevity can be attributed to the importance of the sector's contribution to health care as an additional provider, a pressure group and watchdog, and an innovator. It is also able to focus on minority groups in a way that government cannot, and offers an opportunity for ordinary people to contribute to the care of each other. More generally, there is a case for having an alternative to the State. If we look always to the government for the solution to every health problem, our freedom of action may be undermined and our independence compromised.

Today, greater reliance has been placed on the voluntary sector as successive governments have sought to restrict the role of the State. Like the NHS, this sector, too, has changed. It is now more business-like and likely to operate on the principles of mutual aid and self-help. Using the skills of professionals and the techniques of the market place, it has become adept at fund-raising, selling itself to the public, and retaining the support of a reluctant government.

In considering whether the voluntary sector should take on additional responsibilities, however, account should be taken of a number of factors.

Limitations of voluntary organizations

Resources are a persistent problem for the sector since it relies on private donations and government grants, both of which are likely to dry up in times of economic hardship. Brown (1990) points out that voluntary organizations are the first to be cut back by a local authority under pressure. Less easily explained, but just as devastating, is the paradox that, when governments sought to cut taxation and reduce public spending, people's willingness to give voluntarily diminished.

There is no evidence to support the view that, even where they work well, voluntary organizations are better than statutory ones in terms of cost, efficiency or competence. Despite being increasingly professionalized, their heavy reliance on volunteers raises questions of competence, standards and codes of practice. Selection and training of volunteers are problematic, as is ensuring that they operate on all fronts (volunteers generally have a preference for service-giving rather than administration and clerical work).

As the line between the statutory and voluntary sectors has become blurred, and many voluntary organizations have been drawn into closer and more formal relationships with public services, so their ability to act independently as pressure groups and critics of the State or as courageous innovators, has been impaired. Many voluntary organizations are so large and remote that they are indistinguishable in practice from statutory services and, therefore, also fail to promote voluntarism. At the same time, because they have their own goals and priorities, voluntary organizations can distort the public agenda.

The altruism expressed through the voluntary sector may not be quite what it appears. People who give of their time may do so because they have too much of it on their hands; the unemployed and early retired might prefer to be in paid work. Giving may serve to ease the guilt of those who know they are better off than others, or to thank carers for past care or services yet to come. There is also considerable pressure on people to contribute, with sophisticated marketing techniques, telethons, and so on, being employed to persuade the reluctant. In other words, voluntary work is driven by utilitarianism – the Benthamite calculation that the pain of parting with money is outweighed by the benefits of giving. Inevitably, this has produced inequality within the sector resulting from people's inclination to donate to those causes of which they approve and consistently neglect others.

By the same token, those receiving care from voluntary organizations are supplicants, with no right to receive and to whom the carers are not accountable. Moreover, they are likely to be among the most vulnerable members of society, more, rather than less, in need of the protection that care, guaranteed by the State, offers.

Bearing in mind these factors, it seems clear that voluntary intervention is more appropriate in some areas than others. A universal framework of health care is essential to ensure eligibility, the right to service and political accountability, even if, after that, diversity is felt to be a good thing. Attempts at wholesale substitution of voluntary sector services for public services would be quite unrealistic. The voluntary sector is not in a position to undertake such a major shift (Mayo 1994, p. 41).

Commercialism

The commercial sector has always played a part in health care in Britain, despite the existence of the universal, comprehensive NHS. As indicated in Chapter 3, after 1948 the commercial sector continued to provide both clinical and ancillary services, to offer insurance for the private funding of health care, and to act as a major supplier of health care goods.

A minor player in the early years, the commercial sector's role began to expand from the 1970s and, under the determined hand of Margaret Thatcher, there were explicit moves, such as tax incentives, to stimulate the private sector. As a result, BUPA, the market leader in private health insurance, flourished and American medical insurance companies enlarged their UK operations. In 1976, private hospitals provided 3,500 beds. Ten years later, this figure had reached 10,000 (Small 1989, p. 109). Between 1973 and 1980 expenditure increases for the NHS and the private sector were broadly comparable, whereas between 1980 and 1997 expenditure on the private sector increased at three times the rate in the NHS (OHE 2000). The rise was generally in acute care and outpatient surgery, where costs were relatively low and profits high. But other areas, slower off the mark, such as provision of residential care for the elderly, chronically ill, and people with physical disabilities, and counselling, also began to expand. After 1997 this rate of growth of the private sector, relative to that of the NHS, slowed.

The consultants' contract was modified in the 1980s, permitting them to earn up to 10 per cent of their NHS income privately, which enabled many to take on such work for the first time. Compulsory competitive tendering for ancillary services and the internal market offered further scope for the private sector, as did the higher profile for health promotion; a great deal of health screening came to be provided commercially. Public institutions were officially encouraged to purchase private sector services, and many did so in order to reduce waiting lists. So, paradoxically, private health care was increasingly funded by public money. Conversely, private clinics could hire NHS equipment (see Chapter 6).

Even after 1997, despite the slowing of growth and the proposal to restrict the rights of newly appointed consultants to work privately, the place of the private sector working in tandem with the NHS was endorsed rather than undermined. The PFI was expanded and the Concordat was signed with the Independent Healthcare Association, which pointed out that the private sector delivered, for example, 20 per cent of acute mental health provision, 55 per cent of medium-secure care, and more residential care than the NHS and local authorities combined (Rathfelder 2000).

Nature of the commercial sector

Table 8.1 illustrates that the commercial sector constitutes organizations that are privately owned and allocate goods and services on the basis of willingness and ability to pay. It operates within a market context in which competition between providers and corresponding choice for consumers are central elements. The commercial organizations are funded through the payment of private fees and charges, and must generate enough income to stay in business.

As a result, those responsible for such organizations have narrower, more clear-cut goals than their public sector counterparts. They have to outdo competitors by maintaining or increasing market share in order to make a profit. Broader social goals do not have to be addressed. In maximizing profit, producers are freer from legal and political constraints than their NHS colleagues, but they must be responsive to customers and accountable to shareholders. 'In the private sector there is a direct relationship between commercial success – as measured by profitability and market share – and the standard of customer service' (Lawton and Rose 1994, p. 7).

The business environment is likely to militate against openness and collaboration and to foster instead a culture of secrecy. Within this context, however, commercial managers:

- can take a long-term view on investment
- have more discretion in decision-making
- have the freedom to take risks.

In the mixed economy of health, however, the commercial sector has recognized that, if it is to be successful in the long term, it has to be sensitive to social goals and take some account of health needs as well as demands.

The case for the commercial sector

Some of the arguments used in support of the market are that it serves to:

- extend consumer choice
- reduce waiting lists
- increase efficiency
- improve the costing and pricing of treatments
- inject new ideas.

But these arguments are not accepted unequivocally. Some consumers may have more choice about which doctor to see or which hospital to attend, but they lack the information and expertise to make informed choices. Poorer consumers will have no choice at all. Variety may facilitate choice, but it can also mean inequality.

With respect to efficiency, there is little evidence to support the view that the commercial sector is any better than the public. Private health care markets are not efficient, bed occupancy rates tend to be lower and administrative costs higher (Baggott 1998).

Moreover, attempts to achieve a national service based on a consistent and coherent strategy are likely to be thwarted. The experience of other countries suggests that health care systems dominated by the commercial sector tend to be fragmented, poorly planned and badly co-ordinated. 'The market is the denial of any form of communal planning, producing outcomes which are the result of a myriad of small decisions made by individuals having no thought for the well-being of one another' (Kingdom 1992, p. 57).

Inequalities in health care (see Chapter 7) are likely to be exacerbated. The link between poverty and ill health means that those most in need are least able to pay and insurance companies tend to select for cover those who represent the least financial risk, in other words, the most healthy. In the USA, 16 per cent of the population is uninsured (Baggott 1998; Wall 1996). Thus, the principle of universality is compromised.

Monitoring quality in the private sector is also a challenge. 'Private hospitals have not been subject to inspection by community health councils or subject to any complaints procedure' (Rathfelder 2000).

Although it is always difficult to demonstrate a link between health care activities and health outcomes, the evidence suggests that the commercial approach fares no better than the public. The USA spends twice as much as the UK on health care, yet the infant mortality rate is higher and male life expectancy lower. There is also evidence of unnecessary surgery and over-doctoring. In Britain, as dental and ophthalmic charges have risen, so too have fears that reduced use of services will result in less early detection and treatment of serious conditions such as oral cancer and glaucoma.

There is a view that the expansion of the private sector may be reaching its limits, and it has its own problems of:

- cut-throat competition
- over-capacity
- conflicts between insurers and private hospitals over the pricing of operations and reimbursement of fees
- business failures
- competition from powerful NHS Trusts.

Indeed, it could well be that the private sector has as much to gain from the Concordat as does the NHS.

Is a synthesis possible?

In planning for health care in the twenty-first century, it may be possible to harness the competition that has occurred both among Trusts and between Trusts and private providers, with collaboration and strategic planning, thus obtaining the benefits of both.

> The fundamental principle of the NHS is that care should be provided when it is needed without charge to the patient, not that it should be provided by the public sector. If we could get more health gain for less cost by contracting all NHS services to the private sector then we should do it.
>
> (Rathfelder 2000)

However, this welfare pluralist argument is not accepted by everyone. The sectors do not automatically substitute or compensate for each other. Their cultures are distinct and their goals and motives differ. Shifting from one sector to another has implications for the nature of the service across the board. There are also important considerations with respect to the staff who work in the services. Competition has forced down the wages of some of the lowest paid workers (Baggott 1998), and gender inequalities are enlarged both as a consequence of this and because of the heavy burden that women bear in the voluntary sector.

A long-standing misgiving about the mixed economy of health is that the private sector draws resources away from the NHS, indeed, that the NHS has subsidized the private sector through, for example, the private/agency work undertaken by NHS-trained consultants and nurses.

A further implication of the co-existence of the private and public sectors in health care is the danger of a two-tier system emerging in Britain as in the USA, for example, privately insured patients are able to queue-jump and receive preferential treatment. Jones (1994) believes that this situation is likely to get worse, especially regarding access to non-urgent treatment. Baggott (1998), on the other hand, suggests that a crude dichotomy of this kind is less likely than variations in the quality of services both within and between public and private sectors.

Two points seem clear. First, a retreat from a mixed economy of health care is unlikely. Second, if such an approach is to be successful, it requires a strong government to ensure that collective responsibility for the health of the nation is not lost.

Key points

- There has always been a mixed economy of health care, with both public and private ownership of services, and eligibility on the basis of both ability to pay and need.
- The visibility and influence of the various sectors have fluctuated over the years but since the early 1980s the dominance of the public sector has been called into question.
- The different sectors are founded on different cultures and a different set of motives but, as the ideological context has changed, so the distinction between them has become less clear.
- Since the early 1980s the public sector has been subjected to an uncompromising drive to take on the enterprise culture; the voluntary sector has also become more business-like. The commercial sector, relatively new to the business of health care in Britain, has come gradually to recognize the complexity and constraints associated with the provision of health care.
- The welfare pluralist argument is that it does not matter which sector provides services as long as people get what they need.
- A revival of voluntarism is appealing on moral grounds, offering, as it does, an alternative to State monopoly, while the commercial influence is welcomed for its propensity to generate greater efficiency and concern for the use of scarce resources.
- The future of health care is likely to be based on the involvement of all the sectors and, while there are dangers in assuming interchangeability, there are also opportunities for a synthesis of the best of all worlds.

Guide to further reading

For a good discussion of the nature of the public sector and the changes to which it has been subject over the past twenty-five years, S. Ranson and J. Stewart's (1994) *Management for the Public Domain*, London: St. Martin's Press, is a sound starting point.

The final chapter of L.J. Jones's (1994) *The Social Context of Health and Health Work*, London: Macmillan, discusses issues relevant to the questions raised in this chapter. These include: the crisis in welfare, market principles in health care, accountability, evaluation and the shift from professional autonomy to managerial control.

For its combination of clarity and erudition, R. Klein's (1995) *The New Politics of the NHS*, London: Longman, is an essential text. In this context, his chapters on value for money and the future are the most relevant.

For a broad-based, provocative and stimulating discussion of the roles of the State, market and voluntary sector, J. Kingdom's (1992) *No Such Thing as Society*, Buckingham: Open University Press, provides a lively and accessible read. In arguing that there is such a thing as society, and that political structures which enshrine communal values are essential, he engages and challenges the reader.

Chapter 9
Realigning the system
Towards a primary care-led NHS

OUTLINE
Health care activities can be classed according to various
'levels'. Despite a long biomedical tradition, difficulties associated with the establishment of teamwork, professional divisions
and fragmented organizational structures, the balance is now
shifting away from the secondary sector in favour of a higher
profile for primary care. However, there are two contrasting definitions of primary care – the radical approach epitomized by the
Alma Ata Declaration, and the conservative approach which
appeared to be winning the day. Developments since the end of
the twentieth century, however, suggest that, although slow,
progress towards a genuine re-alignment of the health care
system is in train.

Introduction

Simultaneously with the growth of the mixed economy of health
has been a shift of emphasis away from secondary in favour of primary care. Although separate, the two trends are not entirely
unrelated, stemming as they do from both practical concerns relating to the allocation of resources, and ideological issues to do with
the disposition of power and the principles which should govern
modern health care.

In order to understand exactly what such a shift involves, it is
important to define the levels of health care, namely, self-care, primary, secondary and tertiary. This provides a framework in which
it is possible to analyse the distribution of resources and power in
the health care system and to identify trends.

Self-care refers to any actions taken by individuals to look after
themselves, possibly with help and support from family and friends,

and using medication and appliances bought over the counter. When this proves wanting, primary care will be called into action. Primary care has been described as:

> the point of entry for individuals to [formally provided] health care services, involving functions of assessment and of mobilisation and co-ordination of further medical services; and . . . personal, continuing and long-term care for individuals and families in a local community.
>
> (Brearley *et al.* 1978, p. 66)

Because of the range of health care activities involved and their geographic dispersal, they are delivered by a variety of professionals, among whom the GP has been a central figure.

Secondary care refers to the sophisticated and costly specialist services provided, by and large, in hospitals, which are needed only by a minority of people at any one time. Hospitals deal exclusively with those already defined as being ill. For those who have to stay in hospital, secondary care is institutionally based and continuous and, therefore, more expensive. By contrast, community-based care is partial and intermittent and it is mainly for this reason that it is cheaper. Tertiary care is the term used to describe the super-specialist and intensive care services available only at certain hospitals. Care at this level involves state-of-the-art technology and tends to be very expensive.

The growing awareness of the limitations of secondary and tertiary care, their cost and the difficulty of containing that cost (see, for example, Petchey 1996, Wall 1996) have been strong incentives behind the shift to the primary sector. This has meant greater emphasis on low-tech, preventive measures and undertaking in the community techniques once carried out in hospital (e.g. diagnostic tests, minor surgery, post-operative care and the management of chronic diseases). These moves have been facilitated by surgical and pharmacological developments which enable more conditions to be treated in the community and, where hospital admission is required, to reduce the length of stay. The growing popularity of alternative approaches such as self-help also facilitate this shift of emphasis.

Demographic and epidemiological trends have served to heighten concerns about secondary care. The 'greying' of the population and corresponding growth in the incidence of chronic conditions and disabilities have contributed to spiralling costs and increased the numbers of people for whom care in community settings is most appropriate. The erosion of professional power which has been a consequence of government welfare policies since the early 1980s (see Chapter 5) has also provided a suitable backcloth for a shift of emphasis towards primary care.

And yet while such a change of approach had wide appeal, there was little consensus regarding the adoption of a strategy to under-pin reform and, consequently, practical developments were piecemeal and slow.

The biomedical legacy

The dominance of the secondary sector is related to the fact that the NHS is a health care system deeply rooted in a biomedical model of health and health care (see Table 9.1), defining health narrowly and more interested in treating sickness than in promoting health.

The logic of the biomedical model means that primary care has been conceived largely in terms of its relationship with the sec-ondary sector, merely the first step on the road to cure. For this reason and because it is generally less glamorous, it has been accorded a relatively low status within the health care system. This was buoyed up by the structure and processes of the Service itself and the traditions of professional education.

The tripartite structure, by separating secondary from primary care, and fragmenting primary care, effectively sealed the (subordi-nate) position of those working in the primary sector. Medical science had made its advances in hospital settings; hospitals were the power bases of the consultants and, from being places to avoid, they became the places where heroic medicine took place. Thus, the hospital sector rapidly became the giant of the system, absorbing some 80 per cent of health care resources (Baggott 1998; Wall 1996) and dominating and defining the health care agenda. The primary sector and the professionals staffing it were the David to the hos-pital Goliath.

The health care process meant that the GP dealt with the everyday

Table 9.1 Models of health and illness

	Biomedical	Social
Definition of health	Narrow, negative, opposite of disease	Broad, positive, 'a state of complete physical, social and mental well-being and not merely the absence of disease'
Determinants of health/causes of ill health	Biological causes, origins in germ theory, analogy with body as machine, illness = where a part goes wrong, emphasis on causes of illness	Complex, interacting social, economic, environmental, personal as well as biological factors, emphasis on pre-requisites for health
Approach to health care	Curative, interventionist, clinical research, hospital-based, professionally led, hi-tech, magic bullet, focus on individual	Preventive, promoting/sustaining health, access to prerequisites, focus on population or groups, holistic, inter-disciplinary, inter-agency, epidemiological research, community-based

ailments and anxieties. Many illness episodes did not go past this stage, but GPs also controlled access to the hospitals so there was a sense in which primary care was the precursor to more sophisticated secondary care. GPs were the filterers, signposters, supporters and enablers in a system that was driven, not by them, but by the secondary sector. But all health professionals, whether in the primary or secondary sector, were educated and socialized in the biomedical tradition.

With its apparent ability to apply biomedical sciences to the diagnosis and cure of an ever-lengthening list of human conditions, biomedicine captured the imaginations of the professions and public alike for most of the twentieth century. In many respects, of course, this was justified. Nevertheless, since the mid-1970s there has been growing disquiet regarding both the limitations and the dominance of the biomedical model which cast doubts on its long-term sustainability (Blaxter 1990; Doyal 1981; Macdonald 1993; Stacey 1988).

Cost also became a major focus of concern. Hospital care itself was expensive and most of the increase in demand for health care, in the years after 1948, was centred on the hospitals. Moreover, the cost was difficult to contain. However, there was more to it than just cost. Cures were frequently partial and treatments had side effects (Allsop 1995; Jones 1994; Wall and Owen 1999; Zola 1972). Some 'modern' diseases proved resistant to cure. For the growing numbers of elderly people and those with chronic conditions, disabilities or mental health problems, biomedicine had less to offer. In this context, an increasingly vociferous case was made for adopting the philosophy and principles associated with primary care. (See, for example, Allsop 1986; Ashton and Seymour 1988; Doyal 1981; Macdonald 1993; O'Keefe *et al.* 1992; Townsend and Davidson 1988.)

Were there to be a substantial shift of emphasis towards primary care, it would, in some respects at least, be a step back to simpler, more natural and less invasive forms of care which pre-date modern techniques. But in the past, primary care existed in the absence of these more sophisticated alternatives. Now it would have to take its place in a complex health care system in which secondary care has a well-established hegemony. It is the form that modern primary care takes and the mutual adjustment required between primary care and the wider system, which are of interest.

A declaration of reassessment

One of the major challenges to the continued ascendancy of the secondary sector came from an international conference of the WHO held at Alma Ata in 1977. The conference declared, among other things, that health is a fundamental human right and should be defined in a broad way as a state of complete physical, mental and social well-being and not merely (as in the biomedical model) as the absence of disease or infirmity. Governments have a responsibility for the health of their people and they should aim to achieve a level of health for all that permits them to lead economically and socially productive lives. In pursuing this objective, governments were encouraged to emphasize primary care, address inequalities and ensure that people participate in the planning and implementing of their own health care (WHO 1978).

In response to criticism that the Declaration was broad and idealistic and geared towards the perspectives of developing countries, the global strategy was reformulated into a European Regional Strategy incorporating thirty-eight specific targets for Europe (WHO 1985), one of which made a powerful case for applying the values and principles associated with primary care more broadly. 'By 1990 states should have developed health care systems based on primary care' (WHO 1985: Target twenty-six).

The European strategy received a national focus in Britain with the Health of the Nation (Department of Health 1991a) and the Healthy Cities movement (Ranade 1997). At the same time, the Women's Health Movement (see Chapter 7), although not taking root to the same extent as it did in America, did endorse the need for a change of focus (O'Keefe *et al*. 1992).

A similarly radical concept of primary care was suggested in 1986 in The Report of the Review of Community Nursing, chaired by Cumberlege (DHSS 1986b). Cumberlege argued that community nurses, reorganized as integrated nursing teams on the basis of small neighbourhoods, should have a higher profile within primary care. She sought a more equal relationship between nurses and GPs and written agreements regarding the objectives of the primary care team and the roles of team members. Although the government was not prepared to accept the Report, 'a relatively large number of health authorities responded positively to the concept of neighbourhood nursing' (Ottewill and Wall 1990, p. 433) and by 1988 one-third had developed a Cumberlege-style community nursing service.

In their different ways WHO, the Women's Health Movement and Cumberlege were offering an ambitious definition of primary care and may be said to have paved the way for a fundamental reassessment of modern health care, which, in many respects and by comparison with other countries, Britain was well placed to undertake. The reasons for this are first, there was, in Britain, a well-established and popular NHS in which family practitioner and community health services had a pivotal role. And second, despite difficulties, teamwork had developed in the community and there was fairly wide agreement that the goals associated with a primary care approach should be pursued (Barker 1996). Moreover, the continued urgency of containing costs meant that efforts to restrict the use of hospital services were unlikely to lose momentum.

However, while the effect of the WHO initiatives, the Women's Health Movement and the Cumberlege recommendations was to allow the creation of a culture and a context within which a re-definition of health and health care *could* take place, their agenda may have been too radical. They were not simply seeking to shift the balance of activity more towards the primary sector, but were challenging the idea of primary care as GP-centred and biomedically driven. This was to fly in the face of established working patterns and power relationships, and it raised the question of whether governments would accept such a radical agenda or would take a more cautious and incremental approach to change.

The evolution of primary care in Britain

Throughout the 1980s, primary care was high on the Conservative Government's agenda. Petchey talks of a 'decade when what started as policy flirtation with primary care . . . matured into determined pursuit' (1996, p. 158). The appeal, however, was less its radical potential and more that it appeared to offer a cheaper alternative to hospital services; greater potential for charging; and considerable scope for involving private enterprise.

Initial moves were piecemeal:

- the opticians' monopoly on the supply of spectacles was removed (1984)
- the pharmacists' contract was re-negotiated (1985)
- selected list prescribing was imposed on GPs through the use of financial penalties
- prescription charges were raised year on year

- Family Practitioner Committees were made directly accountable to central government with new responsibilities to plan
  and develop primary care services.

A more systematic approach was heralded in 1986 with the publication of a Green Paper, *Primary Care: An Agenda for Discussion*
(DHSS 1986a) which was followed in 1987 with the White Paper,
*Promoting Better Health: The Government's Programme for
Improving Primary Health Care* (DHSS 1987). Although in the
introduction to the Green Paper primary care was defined as 'all
those services provided outside hospitals' (DHSS 1986a, p. 1), it
dealt in the main with family practitioner services. This could be
partly justified in that the Cumberlege Report, covering community nursing, was published on the same day. However, it probably
also reflected the continuation of the fragmentation referred to
below and signalled the government's intention to secure 'a significant expansion of the role of family practitioners at the
expense of community health services staff' (Ottewill and Wall
1990, p. 417). Two years later, *Working for Patients* (Department
of Health 1989a) contained almost no reference to community
services, which appeared to portend even greater neglect of this
sector in the reformed NHS. Indeed, after the establishment of
fundholding, the number of practice nurses doubled (at the
expense of community nurses), confirming the demise of the
Cumberlege option.

The proposals made in the Green Paper generated such controversy that only a watered-down version was put into practice. GPs
were offered financial rewards for:

- being available for patients for longer hours
- reaching health promotion targets
- undertaking minor surgery
- carrying out health checks on the elderly and children
- producing more information for the public
- working in deprived areas
- participating in postgraduate training.

At the same time eligibility for the basic practice allowance was
made more stringent. More private sector funding for surgery

premises was encouraged. Charges for eye tests and dental check-ups were introduced and cash limits were imposed on the funding of GP practice staff, building and improvements to premises.

Thus were marked out a clear set of principles that were to guide policy-making for the next ten years:

- Cost containment was to be a prime consideration.
- Primary care was to be GP-centred.
- GPs' behaviour was to be controlled by the use of economic incentives and tighter management.
- More private finance would be injected into primary care.
- Patients were to be viewed as customers rather than citizens.

As these measures took hold, there was concern that access to primary care would be adversely affected. The combined effects of targets and budgets meant that the most needy patients were the least welcome, thereby exacerbating the problems faced by many of the most vulnerable members of society. The extension of charging also raised questions about access (Baggott 1998).

The use of financial incentives to secure a shift in GP behaviour proved to be neither universally popular nor unequivocally effective. Incentives can undermine clinical judgement, impose extra work and are sometimes perverse. For example, payments for health checks may have encouraged GPs to spend a disproportionate amount of time with the 'worried well', sometimes referred to as the inverse care law, where the well get more care than the sick. With respect to payment for achieving certain levels of childhood immunization and cervical screening, if GPs could not realistically expect to reach the target, they may as well not try to improve the rate at all, and, for GPs working in deprived or rural areas this was likely to be the case. Moreover, spending on primary care remained difficult to control and rose during the 1980s by more than 3 per cent per year in real terms (Baggott 1998).

Nevertheless, by the early 1990s, the term 'primary care led' had crept into the vocabulary (NHSE 1994, 1996) signalling the evolution of Conservative Government thinking during the decade. Fundholding and the internal market were now in place and the Conservatives appeared optimistic about possible further developments. The creation of self-governing hospital and community

Trusts and experimentation with locality commissioning provided the structural framework for a primary care-led NHS. Purchasing decisions had to be based on a systematic assessment of needs and the logic of this process, in the context of growing understanding of changing demographic and epidemiological patterns and their impact on health care, was likely to lead to a higher profile for low tech community-based services.

However, the internal market was by no means unambiguously helpful in terms of securing a shift towards a primary care approach. Teamwork became the victim both of competition between the providers of health care and of the contract culture. The idea of a social contract between the government and its citizens, so funda-mental to the Alma Ata Declaration, was eclipsed by the pseudo-legal 'contracts' between providers and users characteristic of consumerism. Various charters for patients (Department of Health 1991b; see Chapter 5), refined complaints procedures, and the prac-tice leaflets that GPs were obliged to issue symbolized this shift. In short, although primary care was promoted, it continued to be pred-icated on a narrow, biomedical conception of health and illness.

By the mid-1990s, however, there was something of a modifica-tion of the mood. In 1995 the government launched a debate on the future of primary care, and the report that followed paid more than lip service to a wider understanding of health and health care. It referred to continuous and comprehensive care, properly and professionally co-ordinated in relation to secondary care needs and the needs of local communities, and talked of such '"touchstones" as fairness, accessibility, and responsiveness' (NHSE 1996) – all of which owed more to Alma Ata than to earlier Conservative policies.

October 1996 saw the publication of another White Paper propos-ing pilots on local purchasing; permitting professionals other than doctors to be partners in GP practices; and allowing Trusts to employ salaried GPs (Department of Health 1996a). In 1997, a Primary Care Act allowed pilots of new approaches to GP and dental services, including Personal Medical Services (PMS) con-tracts to supplement the General Medical Services (GMS) contracts under which all GPs worked. PMS opened up the possibility of GP practices tailoring the services they offered more proactively to the needs of the local populations (Department of Health 1997a).

The Labour Government, which came into office in May 1997, was able to capitalize on these developments, and what emerged in its White Paper (Department of Health 1997b) was a modification of the internal market rather than abolition. Even more emphasis was to be placed on the primary care sector as the driving force behind the new NHS. Primary Care Groups (PCGs), led by GPs, were to take over from HAs the commissioning of all but specialist health care services and, ultimately, the provision of all community health services. HAs were given explicit responsibility for the health of the community, and to this end were required to establish Health Improvement Programmes. The aims were to continue to attempt to contain health care costs while, at the same time, through a primary care-led NHS, revitalize values of equality, accessibility and democracy – values resonant both of the Labour Party's own ideological past and that of the NHS.

A primary care-led NHS?

By the 1990s then, arguably, there was an emergent vision of what primary care led meant. Atun, for example, suggested that: 'A Primary Care Led NHS is about developing a health system which has a patient and a community focus as opposed to the historic focus on professionals, structures and services' (Atun 1996, p. 8).

Some twenty years after its original Declaration, the WHO reaffirmed its belief in a primary care-led approach:

> The value of the primary care approach lies in its recognising that health is a central part of human development and not simply the technical process by which health professionals deliver medical care. It is a social and political process that involves people, enabling them to take more control over their own health. It also acknowledges that the health of individuals and communities depends on healthy environments . . . [It requires] a radical reorientation towards the development of health systems whose goal is the improvement of the health and well-being of entire populations. . . . New health services must be proactive and holistic.
>
> (BMJ 1997)

Thus, a primary care-led health care system may be said to be one:

- which is based on a broad definition of health and understanding of illness
- which seeks to emphasize health promotion and illness prevention
- in which needs assessment, priority-setting, service design and delivery, and monitoring, are either done within or driven by the primary sector.

From the 1980s, successive governments have implemented policies for health care that have afforded primary care services a high priority and, in so doing, may be said to have capitalized on the strong family doctor traditions of the NHS. Moreover, it is right to place GPs at the heart of the health care system, given their proximity to patients. Further, the thinking behind the policies has evolved, so that the primary care-led concept itself is now clearer while legislation has been enacted and measures put in place to assist its realization. These may be said to be positive signs of a move in the direction of a primary care-led NHS.

However, it might be too optimistic to expect such a transition to be problem-free. There are complex reasons why change has not been faster and more fundamental and why reform may yet falter. These are to do with:

- differing definitions of primary care
- difficulties surrounding teamwork
- professional issues
- structural matters
- resources.

Differing definitions of primary care

Certainly up to 1997, those committed to the radical concept of primary care, envisaged by the authors of the Alma Ata Declaration, had reason to feel despondent, since it was a narrow definition of primary care that underpinned government policy. Petchey questioned 'the extent to which UK primary care policy genuinely embodies the principles underlying the model of PHC advocated by the WHO' (1996, p. 167) and argued that:

> Attempts to develop PHC in . . . the UK have been hindered by identification of primary health care with primary medical care, and the equation of care with services . . . or even as care delivered by GPs. This has diverted attention from health promotion to disease prevention and treatment, ignored community participation in health, and substituted a narrow, biomedical model of illness and its causation for a broader, multisectoral approach to health.
>
> (ibid., pp. 167–8)

Furthermore, primary care was still seen chiefly as a cost-cutting exercise through which the demand for secondary services would be controlled and so the overall costs of health care contained. Not surprisingly in this context, the commitment of professionals necessary to expedite a genuine change of emphasis was unlikely. While there is now some evidence that cost-cutting has become a lower priority and that health and health care are being defined more broadly with the implications for a broader and more flexible health care system coming to be recognized (that is, a move towards the right-hand side of the model shown in Table 9.1), such a culture change will be long in taking root.

Difficulties surrounding teamwork

Central to both the idea and delivery of a primary care-led system is teamwork. The primary health care team has its roots in the growth of general practice as a profession in the nineteenth century and the employment of nurses by GPs for which, after 1965, they received financial incentives. In some cases this developed into 'attachment' schemes where the traditional master/handmaiden relationship between the doctor and nurse began to give way to one based on a greater degree of equality as community nurses became more professionally confident and secure. Other health care professionals were gradually included in the team, reflecting the growing complexity of medicine and the arguments in favour of a holistic approach. But these developments were reversed in the

1980s with fundholding and the idea of general practices as small businesses employing nursing and other ancillary staff. Notwithstanding the introduction of PCG/Ts and PMS, there are still obstacles in the path of genuinely collaborative teamwork between health care professionals.

Professional issues

Contributing to the slow growth of teamwork have been professional jealousies (Ministry of Health 1959; Hudson 1989; Medical Services Review Committee 1962). The professional culture, in stressing expertise and autonomy, is antithetical to teamwork. Effective teamwork rests on the willingness of each member to recognize and value the expertise of other professionals and to sacrifice a degree of autonomy in the interests of working collaboratively.

GPs, in particular, have been reluctant to do this. They are the descendants of the old apothecaries who traditionally lived above the shop from which they plied their trade. Notwithstanding changes which have brought multi-partner practices working from purpose-built surgeries and health centres, sometimes employing phalanxes of receptionists, nursing staff, practice managers and others, the tradition of independence, autonomy and dominance has continued to inform the approach of the modern GP. Their reluctance to collaborate, particularly beyond the partnership, their poor communications with other groups and general isolation, led Klein to describe general practice as 'an autonomous enclave' (1995, p. 163).

Thus, the GPs' interpretation of teamwork was often out of kilter with the views of other professionals. They certainly assumed they were to be the leaders despite having few of the necessary skills and attributes. In many practices, the reality was of the GPs being in charge, while the other employees were there to help the GP and this tradition was carried forward into PCGs.

Education for general practice was geared towards hospital, curative services; it was not until 1980 that special training was made a compulsory part of the medical syllabus. Thus, GPs have operated consistently within the context of the biomedical approach, taking an individualized view of their patients, only concerned with them when they became sick. In short, GPs were ill prepared for a community-wide perspective and collective stance which are central elements in a primary care-led NHS and this situation did nothing to enhance the principle or practice of primary care.

Measures undertaken in the 1980s and 1990s made matters worse. Rather than seeking to resolve problems associated with professional divisions and rivalry within the primary care team and to establish consensus or unity of purpose, government negotiated separately with the primary care professions and managed to anger them all. Nurses were dismayed by the government's very clear intentions throughout to support a GP-centred approach; with nurses returning to their handmaiden role rather than being viewed as professionals in their own right. Doctors and dentists were unhappy about the new contracts. Later, the assumption that GPs would take the lead role in the emerging PCGs further fuelled resentment on the part of other community health professionals.

So there is a continuing risk that primary care will be dominated by GP-centred biomedicine and that it will remain essentially medical care rather than health care.

Structural matters

Related to teamwork is the structure of the NHS within which primary care was to be delivered. For various historical and political reasons (see Chapters 1 and 2), not only were primary and secondary care divided, but also responsibility was split within the primary sector. On the one hand, there were family practitioners, all of whom were under contract to the government. On the other hand, there were community health services (nurses and professions allied to medicine such as chiropodists and physiotherapists, usually employed by Trusts). Moreover, responsibility for closely related community care services lay with the local authorities. Private health services and voluntary organizations also made a contribution. This fragmentation, together with the independent contractor status of the family practitioners meant that it was difficult to secure either effective collaboration or the holistic approach necessary to underpin a primary care-led system.

Symptomatic of this fragmentation has been the heavily demarcated boundaries between the levels of health care and the difficulties associated with moving between them. Traditionally, decisions about whether or not to cross the boundary between self-care and primary care have been taken by service users rather than professional providers. Primary care services are, thus, reactive and the professionals involved have little control over the nature and extent of demand for them. Nevertheless, there are important exceptions to this, such as dental check-ups, eye tests, screening services, health promotion campaigns, school medicals, home visits by health visitors and vaccination and immunization programmes for children. And so a proactive role for primary care professionals has become more common, and one to which they have become more accustomed, in recent years.

The boundary between primary and secondary care is patrolled by the GP who acts as the gatekeeper, controlling access to expensive secondary care through the process of referral. Although a long-standing practice and one which is found in many other developed health care systems, there are doubts about its efficacy in terms both of the appropriateness of referrals and consistency between GPs (Health Departments 1989; Office of Health Economics 1990; Petchey 1996).

In view of the relative cost of primary and secondary care, the financial implications of inappropriate referral are considerable and the government has taken the matter very seriously. Under the terms of their contract, GPs were required to provide HAs with information about their referrals and, through the creation of PCG/Ts, have been obliged to become more self-critical with respect to their referral decisions. Referral guidelines have been introduced and, in the longer term, it is probable that professionals other than GPs will be involved (NHS Executive 1996).

A number of problems are associated with the movement of patients back from hospital to the community. Timely and accurate information about patients leaving hospital is not always communicated to the appropriate agencies and professionals. Consequently, clinical functions such as physiotherapy do not necessarily continue uninterrupted when the patient re-enters the community (Victor 1991, p. 119). Ideally, there would be a seamless web of care (Royal Commission on the National Health Service 1979, p. 53). But all too often reality falls short of the ideal.

In addition to the structure of the NHS itself, there is today a growing acceptance that there is no need for it to exist and operate in isolation from the private health care sector, and the Concordat signifies steps towards the breaking down of the wall that previously existed between them. Similarly, PCG/Ts include a built-in local authority contribution, while the Care Trusts announced in 2001 are intended to go beyond collaboration into the territory of integrated provision by local authorities and local PCTs.

In sum, it remains to be seen whether recent initiatives can overcome the long-standing and deeply embedded structural obstacles standing in the way of a primary care-led NHS.

Resources

Finally, in addition to structural problems, there are resource issues. Cost containment, although not such a priority under Labour as it was under Conservative Governments, is likely to remain a goal. Yet, if a primary care-led NHS is to be effective there must be a willingness to invest adequate resources.

Between 1979 and 1991 expenditure on primary care increased in absolute and relative terms to its present level of about one-third of NHS current expenditure. This is hardly surprising given increases in the cost of services and the enhanced role that the sector was being called upon to play. Nevertheless, it was disappointing to governments eager to control spiralling health care costs and who saw primary care as a cheaper option. But the lesson surely is that a more cost-effective NHS is one within which more generous support for primary care produces more cost-containment in other parts of the system.

A primary care-led NHS, if it is realized to its maximum potential, will amount to a fundamental re-ordering of the NHS away from a system based upon biomedicine and towards a more inclusive and holistic understanding of what is meant by health. But there are problems with the term primary care and these are exacerbated when we add the word 'led'. And it is an important word, since it means not simply that there shall be primary care – we have had that since before the NHS – but that the Service shall be driven by the primary care sector.

It remains to be seen whether the changes set in train since 1990 are sufficient to achieve a genuine shift of direction for the NHS and, if so, whether this proves a sound way of addressing the challenges of health care in the twenty-first century.

Key points

- A distinction can be made between different levels of health care, namely, self-care, primary, secondary and tertiary.
- In Britain, as in most western nations, the secondary and tertiary sectors have dominated the health care system in terms of both resources and power.
- Since the late 1970s there has been a groundswell of opinion in favour of shifting the balance towards the primary sector and applying the principles of a primary care approach more generally within the health care system.
- A review of the evolution of primary care in Britain revealed that GPs have always played a key role in the NHS but professional divisions, organizational fragmentation and resource problems restricted the development of a true primary care-centred system, thus, policies of successive governments from the late 1970s have been equivocal.
- Primary care can be defined narrowly as centring on the GP and adopting a traditionally biomedical approach, or more broadly incorporating other professionals and taking a more proactive stance in relation to the local population.

Guide to further reading

For a comprehensive approach to primary care, N. Boaden's (1997) *Primary Care: Making Connections*, Buckingham: Open University Press, is a good starting point. There is a good discussion of the history of primary care, current organization and management, the fragmented nature of professions and the politics of primary care. Recommendations are made about new forms of organization and the development of the professions involved.

G. Meads (1996) *A Primary Care-Led NHS*, London: Financial Times Healthcare, is a manual for managers responsible for delivering a primary care-led NHS. It aims to provide a step-by-step, practical guide to every aspect of primary care management from the meaning of policy to monitoring its implementation.

For another 'practical' book but of a different order, see T. Rathwell *et al.* (1995) *Tipping the Balance Towards Primary Health Care*, Hampshire: Avebury, which describes a project of the same title. There are three sub-themes: managing decentralization; indicators for resource allocation and monitoring; and community participation and skills development. These themes are illustrated by detailed case studies of primary care projects in various countries.

Chapter 9 of R. Baggott's (1998) *Health and Health Care in Britain*, Basingstoke: St. Martin's Press, is worth reading for its succinct but comprehensive coverage of many of the main issues.

G. Moon and N. North (2000) *Policy and Place: General Medical Practice in the UK*, Basingstoke: Macmillan, examines general practice within a health policy context. It explores the impact of recent reforms and their implications for general practice in the future.

Chapter 10
Promoting health and preventing illness

OUTLINE
Linked to the higher profile for primary care is the concern to be more proactive in health promotion and illness prevention. Health promotion may take the form of individualist or collectivist strategies, and illness prevention can be at primary, secondary or tertiary level. Government policy has been consistently concerned to support health promotion and illness prevention but has been equivocal about which approach to adopt. This ambiguity can be better understood by exploring the issues surrounding this area of health care: logistical problems, socio-political factors and moral questions.

Introduction

A primary care approach puts its main emphasis on promoting health and preventing illness, which is self-evidently preferable to curing disease. For the individual, staying healthy is better than falling ill and for society as a whole, spending money on preventing disease is a more constructive use of resources than spending it on curing sick people. However, the soundness of the argument has not been matched by progress in either shifting health care resources towards preventive strategies or effectively reducing preventable disease.

Health promotion

Health promotion includes all action designed to improve the health status of individuals and communities. Though including curative interventions, it differs from the traditional curative approach in a number of important ways:

- Measures are directed at the whole population or groups within it, such as ethnic minorities or school children, rather than at individuals.
- It is as much concerned with the subjective aspects of health (feeling well) as with objective clinical abnormalities (being ill).
- Its goal is to enhance the ability of the individual to participate in social and economic life rather than simply to restore physical functioning.
- Given this broad goal and the wide range of environmental factors now known to affect health, those concerned with health promotion are drawn away from the clinical arena and even from the traditional health care system. Care is more likely to take place in community settings such as the home, school and leisure centre; to involve a wide range of agencies such as academic institutions, voluntary organizations and local authorities, as well as mainstream health care agencies; and to rely on the contributions of a wide range of experts.

Individualist and collectivist strategies

Two distinct strands are discernible within health promotion. First, there are initiatives based on the assumption that people can control their own lives and are responsible for their own health. Once termed health education and designed to inform and persuade rather than compel, these are now more commonly referred to as lifestyle campaigns and aim to encourage healthy behaviour (e.g. low fat diets, safe sex) and discourage unhealthy behaviour (e.g. warning of the dangers of smoking).

Second, there are collectivist strategies, based on the recognition that individuals often have limited control over their lives and that much of the responsibility for health lies with the government. These are usually based in law and seek to remove or restrict individual choice in the interests of promoting health. They include:

- building regulations
- environmental and occupational measures, e.g. pollution controls

- rules governing nutrition and the preparation of food, e.g. school meals, meat inspection, hygiene in marketing, control of additives and contaminants, pasteurization.

A recent variant of this approach is that which seeks to make the healthy choice the easy one. This is sometimes referred to as 'healthy public policy', examples of which are pricing policies in the fields of food, leisure, housing and transport and taxation policies with respect to alcohol and tobacco.

Beattie offers a method of classifying the different approaches, in which he posits two continua: first, the mode of intervention, ranging from authoritative to negotiated and second, the focus of intervention going from individual to collectivist (see Figure 10.1). In this way, various forms of intervention can be classified.

	Authoritative mode of intervention	Negotiated mode of intervention
Individual focus	Cell 1 Lifestyle campaigns	Cell 2 Personal counselling
Collectivist focus	Cell 3 Legislative action	Cell 4 'New' public health

Source: Based on Beattie in Gabe *et al.* (1991)

Figure 10.1   Approaches to health promotion

Taking smoking as an example, strategies in Cell 1 are those based on TV and poster campaigns and warnings on cigarette packets. Cell 2 is one-to-one contact between professional and patient, in which the latter seeks and the former provides help and support in giving up smoking. Cell 3 includes laws relating to advertising tobacco products, smoking in public places and smoking policies in organizations. Cell 4, the 'new public health' approach, is founded on the belief that a community, be it a school, workplace or city, might identify issues associated with smoking and plan its own programme for tackling them. WHO's Healthy Cities initiative is a prime example (1985).

Illness prevention

Although there is considerable overlap between health promotion and illness prevention, the latter is more specific and clinicians have a larger and more clearly defined role. It can take place at three levels: primary, secondary and tertiary.

Primary prevention

Primary prevention is the eradication of the disease agent, resulting in fewer new cases occurring. As with health promotion, some of these measures may be directed at the population at large and are sometimes a statutory requirement. Measures to prevent accidents such as the obligation to wear seat belts and crash helmets; laws relating to drinking and driving; child-proof caps on medicines; and motorway crash barriers are examples of primary prevention; as are vaccination and immunization programmes.

Secondary prevention

Secondary prevention involves early, pre-symptomatic diagnosis of a disease, and the subsequent modification of its natural history. It reduces the number of people suffering from it at a specified time. Specific disease screening (e.g. for breast or cervical cancer; tuberculosis and Down's Syndrome) comes into this category, as do routine surveillance procedures such as:

- antenatal care
- monitoring pre-school and school-age children
- medical examinations on entry to employment and for those in selected occupations, e.g. pilots, train/crane drivers.

Some of these measures have fallen victim to financial constraints within the NHS (Bennett 1997) but there appears to be a growing market for personal health checks in the commercial sector.

Tertiary prevention

The third level of prevention seeks to minimize the effects of an illness or disability. The objective is to return the individual to as full a state of health and fitness as possible. Examples include care for the elderly, the chronically sick, people with disabilities and those suffering from AIDS. It means allocating resources to unglamorous parts of the health and social care system and for research in areas which traditionally have not commanded a large share of the research budget.

Government policy

Although its initial remit was to 'secure improvement in the physical and mental health of the people of England and Wales and the prevention, diagnosis and treatment of illness' (Ministry of Health 1946, pp. 9–10), the NHS's subsequent emphasis on cure rather than prevention led to the charge that it was, in fact, a National Sickness Service (see Chapter 5). By the 1970s, however, the drawbacks of the curative approach were apparent.

- For many conditions, particularly those that are major causes of contemporary morbidity and mortality, such as cancer, cures remained elusive.
- Treatment is often very expensive.
- Many cures were partial and carried risks which Illich (1975) termed 'iatrogenesis' (e.g. addiction to, and the side effects of, prescription drugs).
- The curative approach has made only a limited contribution to improving the health of the population. This has been reflected in part in the ever-growing demand for health services.
- Likewise, it has had a limited impact on the endemic inequalities in health status associated with class, gender and race (see Chapter 7).

In 1976, the government signalled its intention to shift the locus of power within the NHS when it declared that its aim was to encourage HAs to place more emphasis on preventative activities when planning services and resource allocation (DHSS 1976). Three years later, the Royal Commission expressed its 'regret that more emphasis has not been placed in the past on the preventive role of the NHS. This must change if there is to be substantial improvement in health in the future' (Royal Commission on the National Health Service 1979, p. 41).

The climate remained the same during the 1980s. In 1981, the government declared the need for every HA to develop a local strategy of health promotion and illness prevention (DHSS 1981), and in 1987 reaffirmed the need to shift the emphasis from treatment to the promotion of health and the prevention of disease (DHSS 1987). Acheson believed that one of the problems facing the NHS had been that prevention of illness and promotion of healthy lifestyles had been implicit rather than explicit objectives and that responsibility for these had been ill-defined (Acheson 1988). The Public Health Alliance asserted that one of the principles of the 'new' public health movement is that the protection of the public and the prevention of illness should be given priority over costly individual intervention (Public Health Alliance 1988). By the 1990s, the international initiatives, discussed in Chapter 9, had given the arguments added urgency and the government was moved to talk in terms of a key policy objective being 'the need . . . to focus as much on the promotion of good health and the prevention of disease as on the treatment, care and rehabilitation of those who fall ill' (Department of Health 1991a, p. vii). Indeed, the aim of Healthy Sheffield (part of the Healthy Cities project) is to reduce the 'incidence of preventable physical and mental illnesses and disabilities' and to promote 'positive physical and mental well-being' (Healthy Sheffield 1985, p. 4).

Progress, however, has been slow. In 1999 the Labour Government published its White Paper *Saving Lives: Our Healthier Nation*, which stressed the need for a more coherent and concerted approach to reducing avoidable illness (Baggott 2000), and from 1999 HAs and PCG/Ts began to collaborate in the production of HImPs for their local populations. Britain still compares unfavourably with many developed countries for rates of death from coronary heart disease, infant mortality, and alcohol consumption.

Issues

The issues at the heart of health promotion and illness prevention fall under three headings: administrative or logistical problems, socio-political factors and moral or ethical questions.

Administrative problems

The distinction between health promotion and illness prevention, and the different approaches to each, are reflected in uncertainty as to which approach is likely to be most effective in any particular circumstances. For example, should women be exhorted to examine their own breasts, should GPs be encouraged to hold regular well-woman clinics, or should there be a national breast screening programme? Whichever strategy is adopted (and in practice a mixture will usually be apparent), a large number of agencies and professional groups will need to be involved, making collaboration and teamwork more urgent than ever. This is an area in which the NHS has traditionally performed badly (O'Keefe *et al.* 1992; Ottewill and Wall 1990).

Predictably, one of the central administrative issues is the ever-urgent requirement to consider the effective and efficient use of resources. However, the assessment of the relative costs and benefits is not straightforward. In addition to the considerable outlay required in terms of financial resources and professional time and expertise to mount and maintain campaigns, there are a number of hidden costs, which are not always counted, nor, indeed, are they easy to count. Examples of these are:

- the opportunity costs for the NHS
- anxiety for the patient
- potential additional demands if the preventive strategies bring to light undetected need
- where programmes rest on compulsion, the costs associated with enforcement and legitimate exemptions.

There may be few benefits in the short term. Money has to be spent without immediate pay-off and, for the NHS, like most organizations, scarcity of resources has meant a continuing preoccupation with short-term issues rather than investing for the long term. Even in the long term there may be no financial benefits for the NHS. Preventing one particular disease now does not guarantee health but leaves the individual exposed to the 'next hazard'. Indeed, past successes in prolonging life have contributed to the growing numbers of elderly people now making heavy demands on health care resources.

There is a more subtle resource issue here as well. Some of the costs and benefits accrue to the individual and some to society at large. The benefits to an individual being screened for HIV may be very small and the costs very high, but the potential benefit to society at large is enormous in terms of both preventing its spread and collecting vital epidemiological data.

Vaccination and immunization provide another good example of the tension between individual and public benefit. A comprehensive vaccination programme is of unequivocal value to the community at large. For any one individual, however, while there is also benefit in terms of reduced susceptibility to disease, there is also a risk (albeit very small). In truth, therefore, the best situation from the individual's point of view is for everyone else to be vaccinated.

Campaigns to reduce smoking and drinking provide examples of a clear benefit to the individual in terms of improved health and life expectancy, but society at large also gains from reduced passive smoking and fewer accidents resulting from drinking and driving. The cost-benefit equation is complex.

Secondary prevention also generates administrative and logistical problems. First, decisions have to be made regarding whom to screen. Concentrating on a small number may be very effective for them, but has little effect on the health status of the population at large. Indicators can be used but their effectiveness depends on their reliability. For example, age is used as an indicator for breast cancer screening, as the risk of breast cancer is associated with age. However, two-thirds of victims fall outside the age limits for the statutory screening programme (50–64 years). Lowering the age limit has resource implications and is not necessarily the answer as the test is less reliable with younger women.

Second, mechanisms have to be set in place to identify and reach the target population and to monitor the effects of the intervention.

Many people do not respond to invitations for screening and much time and effort has been devoted to ascertaining their reasons and deciding what should and can be done about them.

Third, screening is not a 'one-off', it has to be undertaken regularly. The fact that a woman does not have cervical cancer this year does not mean she will not have it next year. Again, the long-term commitment to a screening programme has resource implications for HAs.

Finally, the collection and use of the information necessary for screening are costly.

Because of these problems, the Department of Health has drawn up protocols to guide those who have to decide whether or not to go ahead with a screening programme. These suggest that a number of factors should be taken into consideration:

- whether it is an important health problem in the sense of causing premature death, loss of productivity, or presenting an unfavourable comparison with other countries
- the extent of knowledge about the cause and natural history of the disease
- the availability of effective and acceptable treatment (HIV screening fails on the former count, and foetal screening often on the latter, since the only 'treatment' available is abortion which is unacceptable to many women)
- the ability and willingness to make resources available for treatment
- the validity and accuracy of screening tests (cervical screening has faltered on this count, as the test has a false negative of up to 20 per cent and the test requires great professional skill and judgement to interpret)
- the cost-effectiveness of the procedure
- agreement on a policy for the management of borderline cases
- ensuring that it is a continuing process with re-testing at intervals determined by the natural history of the disease.

Socio-political factors

A second set of issues impeding progress in promoting health and preventing illness is to be found in the environment in which people live and decisions about health are made – both the immediate NHS environment and the wider social context.

The NHS was created at a time when the biomedical approach dominated. This coloured every aspect of the service. Medical and other clinical professionals were trained and socialized into the biomedical model and non-clinical professional hierarchies came to reflect the kudos attached to curative care. Changing the culture and emphasis of professions and services has not proved easy. The power and prestige of the medical profession are vested in diagnosis and treatment.

A genuine shift of emphasis from cure to prevention requires a willingness to allocate scarce resources to non-urgent and often unglamorous areas. It also means recognizing that the contribution of managers to the success of preventive programmes is equal to that of clinicians; indeed, the boundary between the clinical and the managerial role is unclear. Thus, a change in the relationship and the balance of power between managers and clinicians is required (see Chapter 5).

Much health promotion, particularly that founded on a negotiated mode of intervention (see Figure 10.1), rests on the assumption that people are both able and willing to change their behaviour in the interests of promoting their health. This is to ignore the wider context which, in practice, restricts the control people have over housing, income and working conditions and shapes the personal choices they make about lifestyle.

The poor are consigned to living and working in conditions likely to damage their health and have incomes which restrict their ability to purchase healthy lifestyles. Hilary Graham's influential work on families and health graphically depicts the reality of life for many poor families in which health is but one consideration among many others more immediately and directly concerned with survival. She argues that policies based on the notion of individual choice will frequently fail since

> choice occurs within, and is contoured by, the routines of everyday life. For many families, the limits of choice are narrow and the routines, in consequence, are strict and unbending . . . while change is possible, it involves more than will-power. The conclusion to be drawn . . . is that health

> policies based around responsibility and choice must face the
> material realities . . . [and demonstrate] an awareness of the
> way in which the class structure . . . continue[s] to shape the
> distribution of health resources and responsibilities.
>
> (Graham 1984, p. 188)

Even among those with adequate material resources, behaviour proves difficult to change (Gabe *et al.* 1991). The results of a survey of middle-class families showed that parents and children were in no doubt as to the 'healthy' options (and they were in a position to afford them) but did not always take them (Brackett 1990). Part of the reason for this is that behaviour is guided by attitudes, beliefs and values that are learned and internalized at an early age, reinforced throughout life, and legitimized by the broader socio-political context. The explanations offered by respondents themselves in the above survey were that the 'healthy' options did not fit in with other pressures and commitments in their lives and that their personal preferences directed them towards a less healthy lifestyle. In the case of young people, the need to feel part of the 'in crowd' or to express rebellion are powerful motivators. Financial considerations, stress, boredom and the fact that immediate gratification outweighs future benefits, especially for those whose stake in the future may seem to them very tenuous, all play their part in explaining the persistence of health-damaging behaviour.

Underlying all these factors, however, are the powerful commercial organizations with strong incentives to sell goods and services which damage our health. Governments have been reluctant to cross swords with them, as well, arguably, as to forgo the tax revenues which their products generate. Moreover, there is a genuine tension in a free enterprise economy between the rights of businesses such as tobacco and fast food companies to advertise and sell their products, and the desire of governments to promote health.

Moral questions

A central tenet of the Hippocratic Oath, which forms the basis of the code of medical ethics, is to do the patient no harm. Yet any form of intervention must involve some harm, however small. Because health promotion and illness prevention must involve intervening in the lives of people who are well, it has to be justified more consciously than curative care. Some commentators question the professional's right to intervene in the lives of the healthy, arguing that it is often difficult to justify the infringement of liberty and invasion of privacy involved (Fitzpatrick 2001; Zola 1972). A more conventional view is that intervention is acceptable, on moral grounds, if the incidence of disease and premature death can be reduced without undue invasion. However, this is a treacherous equation. What constitutes undue invasion?

The element of compulsion necessary for many of the programmes founded on an authoritative mode of intervention (see Figure 10.1) is unacceptable to many. Indeed, health promotion has been described as 'a kind of militant wing of public health' (Scriven and Orme 2001, p. 4). The protests against the compulsory wearing of seat belts and crash helmets and the disquiet about fluoridation of water provide evidence of this.

Also, strategies that use persuasion and education tend to be less effective with those at greatest risk and therefore exacerbate inequalities in health. This raises a new set of moral questions.

Some programmes may be more subtle but no less intrusive. The purpose of much intervention is to change people's attitudes and beliefs in order to modify their behaviour. It must, therefore, transgress the moral requirement to respect the person. Moreover, many of the programmes depend upon HAs holding a good deal of personal information about individuals. This raises questions about:

- confidentiality
- ownership and sharing
- whether information collected for one purpose can be used for another
- the use of professional time to collect it.

In 1979, the Royal Commission commented on intrusion as follows:

> To what lengths should society go, to force each one of us to do things which are good for him [*sic*]? In a free society it is

unlikely that we shall be compelled to take exercise or to eat things which are good rather than bad for us except by social pressure. But society can choose to fine those who do not wear seat belts in cars, to fluoridate all drinking water . . . and to tax cigarettes and alcohol punitively. Opponents of such measures argue that they are an unwarrantable intrusion on the freedom of the individual.

(Royal Commission on the
National Health Service 1979, p. 43)

The climate has changed a good deal since 1979, and we have come to accept a higher level of intrusion in our lives. However, the underlying tensions and dilemmas remain much the same.

The decision to intervene in people's lives in a particular manner is informed by certain assumptions regarding responsibility for health and health behaviour. On the whole, the curative approach is morally neutral; few questions are asked about causative factors. The clinician's job is to do whatever is possible to treat the condition. With health promotion and illness prevention it is necessary to make certain assumptions about responsibility and, in a sense, to apportion blame.

There are two broad schools of thought: one blames the victim – the individual who drinks or smokes too much and generally fails to adhere to the exhortations of the health educators. The other takes a more structural view, laying the blame on the economic system for making a profit out of health-damaging goods and on the government for failing to control commerce and allowing conditions to continue in which people feel the need to drink or smoke or lack the incentive to invest in their own health. The individual is an easier target, but has less control over health matters than may be assumed. Commercial enterprises have more control and many believe should be held more responsible than they are, but they are more difficult to hold to account.

What of the impact of prevention? This can be measured only in the medium or long term and only at a societal level. For example, it is impossible to prove that a particular individual would have contracted whooping cough had they not been vaccinated, but it is possible to demonstrate a link between the incidence of the disease and levels of vaccination in a population over a period of time. Thus, many moral questions arising from preventive strategies revolve around the tension between personal freedom and the collective good. Should one person's freedom to smoke in public be curtailed in order to maintain a clean atmosphere? While this particular argument might go in favour of the non-smoking majority, the principle might be less clear-cut with a different example: should the freedom of one person to eat an unhealthy diet be given precedence over the right of the tax payer to keep down the costs of treatment of preventable illness?

Another set of moral questions arises from the adequacy and accuracy of the knowledge about causation upon which strategies are based. This not only affects the likelihood of success, but also the legitimacy of the intervention (Le Fanu 1999). Preventing something from happening implies knowledge of what causes it, yet despite the authoritative nature of much health promotion and illness prevention, the knowledge on which it is based is often incomplete.

Many diseases, particularly those currently the object of preventive strategies, appear to be the result of an interaction between a multitude of factors. While a good deal is known about factors associated with a particular disease ('risk' factors), it is not possible to identify all the components which, when occurring in a particular configuration, inevitably lead to the development of the disease. In other words, risk is not the same as cause. Thus, it is not possible to say that someone who smokes sixty cigarettes a day, has a high fat diet and takes no exercise will have a heart attack. What can be said is that 20 per cent of such people will spend time in a coronary care unit, therefore, the risk for any one individual is 20 per cent. If information is presented to the public in this manner, individuals may be prepared to take the risk rather than change their lifestyle. They may choose to believe that they will be one of the 80 per cent.

The other side of the coin is the danger of raising the expectations of those who do choose to adopt healthy lifestyles and who may then expect to be guaranteed consistently good health and a long life.

There is a further danger, that of focusing on those factors that are most easily controlled or suit one's purposes better. For example, an employer is likely to focus more on the ill effects of lifestyle than stress at work. Similarly, the government is likely to emphasize smoking rather than bad housing as a contributory factor in bronchitis.

In summary, then, whether the incidence of disease and premature death can be reduced without undue invasion in people's lives remains an open question. Moreover, these moral issues, added to the administrative and logistical difficulties and set in the wider socio-political context, make health promotion and illness prevention an exacting area.

The future

It is likely that efforts to shift the emphasis in health care towards a more preventive approach will be maintained. Its benefits may not be measurable in financial terms and may be difficult to measure in human terms. There will be awesome administrative costs, logistical problems and ethical dilemmas. The difficult decisions that will have to be taken should be made in the light of knowledge of these issues and open debate about how to proceed, involving as wide a variety of interests as possible.

Key points

- Health promotion and illness prevention are related to moves to raise the profile of primary care. They embrace a number of different approaches and strategies.
- Since the 1970s governments have tried to shift resources away from cure and towards prevention.
- Logistical and administrative problems, socio-political factors and ethical questions make progress in health promotion and illness prevention a complex area.

Guide to further reading

S. Rodmell and A. Watt's (1987) *The Politics of Health Education: Raising the Issues*, London: Routledge and Kegan Paul, was one of the first books to examine the political implications of health education and to reflect upon the politics inherent in a subject previously thought to be apolitical. It is still very relevant today.

J. Katz, A. Peberdy and J. Douglas's (1997) *Promoting Health: Knowledge and Practice*, London: Macmillan in association with the Open University, explores the meaning of health promotion in the context of the social, economic and cultural factors that affect health. The authors give a good critical review of methods and tackle the thorny questions surrounding the evidence base of health promotion.

J. Naidoo and J. Wills (1994) *Health Promotion: Foundations for Practice*, London: Balliere Tindall, is concerned to set the identification and evaluation of the health promotion role in a broad critical and theoretical perspective and has something to offer all students.

Also interesting is Michael Fitzpatrick's (2001) *The Tyranny of Health*, London: Routledge. The author, a GP, argues that health promotion campaigns are a form of bullying and do more harm than good.

A welcome addition to the literature in this field is R. Baggott (2000) *Public Health: Policy and Politics*, Basingstoke: Macmillan.

Chapter 11

The NHS – fit for the future?

Providing health care in a modern state

During the twentieth century, medicine and the State became allies. Porter talks of 'the socialization of medicine and the medicalization of society', so that medicine 'imperceptibly obtained a place at the table of power' (1997, pp. 634–5; 638). It would be difficult to exaggerate the impact of health care on the lives of the people since 1948, or the part played by the NHS. However, we must recognize that the picture has blemishes. Does medicine sometimes appear to offer, or do we sometimes appear to expect, too much – as long a life as possible, preferably with minimum pain or inconvenience? Have doctors become the high priests of modern society?

Britain at the start of the twenty-first century offers a good standpoint from which to study the strengths and the weaknesses of public health care. The experiment started in 1948 was grandiose – to remove, so far as medical science permitted, as many obstacles as possible to the enjoyment by all the citizens of a reasonably long and healthy life. Results were to be achieved through a collaboration between the clinical professions (who would provide the knowledge and skills) and the State (which would provide the funding and the infrastructure). The experiment succeeded more than it failed but the previous chapters of this book have drawn attention to the main areas where it has left something still to be desired.

We have seen, for example, how the scientific biomedical approach that has characterized the NHS, and which has been responsible for much of its success, has, at the same time, produced a system of health care that concentrates on cure more than on prevention. Moreover, even the cures have not in practice been universally available, since some groups in society have benefited much less than others; the health care actually delivered by the

NHS has not matched the promises made in 1948. The public health movement of the nineteenth century has lost ground to cures based upon specific aetiologies, and if, at the present time it appears to be making this up, it still has some way to go.

The delivery of health care has clearly been beset with problems, whether they arose from the structure of the system, from the absence of a coherent overall strategy, from difficulties in exerting control or imposing direction, or from the entrenched position of the clinical professions. Meanwhile, the cost of care has kept rising, to the point where it has become of serious concern and raises the question whether, as a society, we can continue to try to provide health care that accords with the founding principles.

The story since 1948 is one of almost constant change. The NHS has re-invented itself as new challenges emerged. An ageing population, changing patterns of disease, technological development, fluctuating economic fortunes, concern over public spending and new political ideologies and agendas all have contributed to this moving picture of health care. Although successive governments committed themselves to the founding principles, the academic world is less certain that these principles – universality, comprehensiveness and equity – can be preserved indefinitely (Klein 1995; Powell 1997).

Responding to the challenge

There have been two main types of response to the challenge of providing health care in a modern State. The first, 'sector reform', involves a shift away from the public towards the voluntary and commercial sectors, while attempting to make the public sector operate more commercially. These are the processes of privatization and marketization (see Chapters 3, 6 and 8). These processes have been prompted largely by financial concerns regarding economy and efficiency (see Chapter 4), and a political ideology that places faith in market mechanisms while doubting the ability of public sector organizations to operate at maximum efficiency. The most recent manifestations of this attitude are to be found in the continuation and extension of the PFI and the establishment of the Concordat.

The second type consists of efforts to reduce the dominance of secondary care and promote a greater reliance on primary care (see Chapter 9). This means challenging the centrality of the (expensive) curative, hospital-based approach in favour of the (cheaper) community. This involves focusing more on health promotion and illness prevention, founded on a social model of health care informed by the principles of the Declaration of Alma Ata (1978), and elaborated upon in subsequent WHO initiatives as well as government White Papers. Champions of these initiatives have been instrumental in enhancing the status of primary care and contributing to the renaissance of public health. They have helped legitimize the concept of community participation in setting the health care agenda, designing services and modes of delivery and in holding health care professionals accountable. In other words, it is an approach that seeks to apply a holistic set of principles to the whole of the health care system whether it is primary or secondary; preventive or curative; hospital based or located in community settings. These moves were discussed in Chapters 9 and 10. Both sets of responses are well established and unlikely to be reversed.

A new NHS?

It is against this background that the Labour Government published the White Paper *The new NHS* at the end of 1997 (Department of Health 1997b), followed a little over two years later by *The NHS Plan* (Department of Health 2000b). Taken together, along with other documents, measures and ministerial pronouncements, they give a picture of an NHS which, it is claimed, will deliver a generally higher standard of health care which corresponds more closely to the actual needs of the population and which is premised upon a view of sickness and health extending beyond the strictly biomedical so as to take in social and environmental factors.

The changes encompass both processes and structures. In terms of process, the watchword appears to be collaboration, between different parts of the NHS such as primary and secondary care organizations, and between the NHS and local authority departments. The front-line NHS and local authorities have always employed a local population focus, but they have done so from different perspectives – the one essentially medical, the other primarily social. Collaboration in the new context is intended to embed what might be termed a socio-medical perspective, particularly through the medium of Care Trusts (not to be confused with PCTs) which will bring together local authority and NHS staff for the commissioning and provision of integrated services for particular client groups such as the elderly.

Structurally the changes appear to push in two different directions – decentralizing and centralizing – at the same time. Decentralization is to be found in the establishment from 1999 of PCGs, which by 2004 will have given way to a national network of PCTs controlling between them 75 per cent of the total NHS budget. At the same time, the number of HAs will have been cut by two-thirds. The thirty or so remaining HAs, covering average populations of 1.5 million, are intended to function as strategic bodies rather than as providers of health care, and the present Regional Offices, together with the NHS Executive, will disappear. In the words of Secretary of State Alan Milburn, 'we intend to shift the centre of gravity to the NHS frontline' (Milburn 2001). The picture, then, is of PCTs as the driving force, operating under a lightweight carapace provided by the strategic HAs and, at more of a distance, the Department of Health.

And yet NHS organizations now enjoy the attentions of such bodies as NICE, the Health Improvement Commission (CHImP), the Modernisation Agency and the National Clinical Assessment Authority (NCAA), as well as the imperatives of clinical governance, life-long learning and compulsory National Service Frameworks (NSFs), each of which is a part of a process of setting and monitoring the implementation of national standards. The laudable-sounding aim is to universalize the best although, as Klein (2001) points out, that is actually an oxymoron.

The first government budget of the new millennium, in March 2000, announced very substantial real term increases for the NHS. But increased resources do not necessarily equate with increased freedom. It is perfectly possible to increase funding but at the same time to keep a closer watch on and direction over how the money is spent. In the past politicians have found it almost impossible to direct the NHS with any degree of detail. With the internal market they stopped trying and opted instead for a strategy of re-writing the rules of the game so that, as they hoped, the NHS would have no option but to operate in the way they wished. Today, measures taken since the demise of the internal market, although different in detail, appear to be following the same strategy.

Decentralizing measures are certainly being put into place, but within a larger framework which is intended to ensure that the decentralized powers are used correctly. If this amounts to guided decentralization, this too might be an oxymoron. Klein (2001) uses the analogy of a corset – an article of clothing which, under cover and unseen, pushed and pulled a woman into the right shape before allowing her to go on about the business of being a woman.

And so the cosmology of the NHS is changing (see Figure 11.1). In its very early days, the universe in which we live only really began to come alive when stars switched themselves on. Stars coalesced into galaxies revolving around a central point. And then the whole thing is held together by gravity, which links every particle with every other particle. But the stars are the essential feature; without stars, no galaxy.

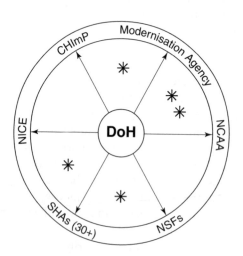

✳   PCT (200+)

DoH = Department of Health

Figure 11.1   The cosmology of the new NHS

In the galaxy of the NHS the Department of Health is at the centre (and might, if it is too heavy-handed, come to be seen as something of a black hole, gobbling up the autonomy of the PCTs). Circling around the galaxy are such bodies and imperatives as NICE, CHImP, the Modernisation Agency, NSFs, the NCAA and Strategic HAs. These provide the gravity that holds the whole thing together. But it is the PCTs that are coming to life as stars, circled by their own solar systems (not shown in the diagram) of organizations with which they collaborate to provide the health care needed in their particular part of the galaxy.

A great deal of bargaining and negotiation, as well as administrative and financial preparation, were needed to turn the words of the 1946 Act into the reality of the NHS in 1948. The task now is to turn the new NHS into reality. The pressures to which the NHS has been subjected in recent years raises concerns about the effect on those who, at the end of the day, deliver the health care. It still remains to be seen whether the public health care system is to receive a shot in the arm or a nail in the coffin, whether the centre will allow the stars to shine.

Glossary

Biomedical approach: the approach to illness and health care which utilizes the scientific approach of deductive reasoning, using symptom observation to arrive at a diagnosis of the individual patient's condition; this approach is prevalent in Western medicine and has been responsible for many of its most noteworthy advances whilst, at the same time, tending to neglect less easily observed factors from, for example, the patient's environment.

British Medical Association (BMA): the chief representative organization for British doctors, to which three-quarters of practising doctors belong; originally established in 1832, it has worked effectively as both a pressure group and a trade union, influencing the shape of the NHS and health policy over many years.

Clinical autonomy: the right of clinical professionals (particularly doctors) to exercise their skills and judgement in the diagnosis and treatment of illness free from outside direction.

Clinician: a professionally qualified health worker with direct responsibility for patient care.

Compulsory competitive tendering: government imposed requirements that private sector organizations be invited to tender for work presently undertaken within the public sector, e.g. hospital cleaning and laundry services; the expectation was that private sector organizations would be cheaper, and would either win the contracts or oblige the public sector to reduce its costs.

Department of Health: the central government department responsible for determining policy and priorities and allocating resources to the NHS and Health Authorities.

Evidence-based medicine (EBM): approach to the allocation of health care resources based upon the systematic assessment of the effectiveness of different interventions.

Founding values: the principles which guided the creation of the National Health Service, i.e. that it should be comprehensive (covering all types of health care), universal (including the whole population), free at the point of use (being funded from general taxation), and equally accessible to everyone.

Fundholding: a central feature of the internal market (q.v.) whereby GPs were given their own practice budgets.

General Medical Council (GMC): created by the Medical Act of 1858, the Council acts as the regulatory and disciplinary body for the medical profession, oversees medical education investigates doctors.

Health Authorities: within the NHS, the bodies responsible for co-ordinating health service provision over a given geographical area.

Internal market: sometimes described as a quasi-market, the classification of agencies within the NHS (e.g. GP practices, Health Authorities, hospitals) as either purchasers or providers of health care, with the intention of generating competition and increasing efficiency; an attempt, therefore, to simulate the competitive commercial sector within the NHS.

Managed competition: an alternative term for the internal market, which stresses the importance of managing competition particularly in the context of health care.

Marketization: the introduction of a more commercial culture into health care provision, e.g. seeing patients as customers; marketization, whilst clearly linked to the internal market concept, is broader.

Medical audit: the systematic measurement of clinicians' performance against agreed standards, with a view to improving care.

Medical Officer of Health (MOH)/Director of Public Health: the office of MOH was created in 1848, the holder being responsible for the health of the public and for overseeing community health services within a local authority area; MOHs disappeared in 1974, the role re-emerging as Director of Public Health, this time within Health Authorities, after the 1988 Acheson Report.

Mixed economy/welfare pluralism: pluralism as a model of political activity recognizes the existence of competing actors in the political arena; similarly, welfare pluralism suggests the existence of a number of alternative sources of health care, i.e. public, commercial and informal. A mixed economy of health is one, which acknowledges the contribution of each of these sectors.

National Health Service Executive: in response to the Griffiths Report highlighting the importance of the management function, the NHS Executive was established in 1989 to be responsible for the day-to-day management of the NHS within the policy guidelines laid down by the government; reabsorbed into the Department of Health in 2001.

NHS Trusts: within the context of the internal market, they are hospitals or community units given a considerable degree of financial and managerial independence.

Royal Colleges: the royal medical colleges (such as the Royal College of Surgeons founded in the eighteenth century, and the Royal College of Physicians founded in the sixteenth, as well as the more recent ones such as the Royal College of General Practitioners and the Royal College of Nursing) are responsible for the education, training and registration of medical specialists; from time to time they also become involved in public issues relating to health care.

World Health Organization (WHO): founded in 1948 as an international organization to promote improved health world-wide.

References

Abercrombie, N. and Warde, A. (1995) *Contemporary British Society*, 2nd edn, Cambridge: Polity Press.

Abrams, P. (1978) *Neighbourhood Care and Social Policy*, Berkhamstead: Volunteer Centre.

Acheson Report (1988) *Public Health in England: The Report of the Committee of Enquiry into the Future Development of the Public Health Function*, Cm 289, London: HMSO.

Addison, P. (1994) *The Road to 1945*, rev. edn, London: Pimlico.

Adonis, A. and Pollard, S. (1997) *Class Act: Myth of Britain's Classless Society*, London: Hamilton (Hamish) Ltd.

Allsop, J. (1984) *Health Policy and the NHS*, London: Longman.

Allsop, J. (1986) 'Primary health care – the politics of change', *Journal of Social Policy* vol. 15, part 4, pp. 489–96.

Allsop, J. (1995) *Health Policy and the NHS, Towards 2000*, 2nd edn, London: Longman.

Annandale, E. and Hunt, K. (eds) (1999) *Gender Inequalities in Health*, Milton Keynes: Open University Press.

Ashton, J. and Seymour, H. (1988) *The New Public Health*, Buckingham: Open University Press.

Atun, R. (1996) 'Primary Care-Led NHS', *Clinicians in Management*, vol. 5, no. 4, pp. 8–11.

Baggott, R. (1998) *Health and Health Care in Britain*, Basingstoke: St. Martin's Press.

Baggott, R. (2000) *Public Health: Policy and Politics*, Basingstoke: Macmillan.

Bagilhole, B. (1997) *Equal Opportunities and Social Policy*, London: Longman.

Baldock, J. and Ungerson, C. (1991) 'What d'ya want if you don' want money?: a feminist critique of paid volunteering', in M. Maclean and D. Groves (eds) *Women's Issues in Social Policy*, London: Routledge.

Barker, C. (1996) *The Health Care Policy Process*, London: Sage Publications.

Barnes, C. and Cox, D. (1997) 'Patients, power and policy: NHS management reforms and consumer empowerment', in K. Isaac-Henry, C. Painter and C. Barnes (eds) *Management in the Public Sector*, 2nd edn, London: International Thomson Business Press.

Bennett, F. (1997) 'Social policy digest', *Journal of Social Policy*, vol. 6, part 2, p. 248.

Beveridge, W. (1942) *Social Insurance and Allied Services*, Cmd 6404, November, London: HMSO.

Bilton, T., Bonnett, K., Jones, P., Stanworth, M., Sheard, K. and Webster, A. (1990) *Introductory Sociology*, 2nd edn, London: Macmillan.

Blaxter, M. (1990) *Health and Lifestyles*, London: Tavistock.

BMJ (1997) *Health Care Systems for the 21st Century* (7th Consultative Committee on Primary Care Systems for the 21st Century), 314: 1407, 10 May.

Boaden, N. (1997) *Primary Care: Making Connections*, Buckingham: Open University Press.

Brackett, K. (1990) 'Image and reality: health enhancing behaviour in middle class families', *Health Education Journal*, vol. 49, no. 3, pp. 61–3.

Brearley, P., Gibbons, J., Miles, A., Topliss, E. and Woods, G. (1978) *The Social Context of Health Care*, London: Basil Blackwell and Martin Robertson.

Brown, M. (1990) *Introduction to Social Administration in Britain*, 7th edn, London: Hutchinson.

Buchan, J. (2000) 'Abroad minded', *Health Service Journal*, 6 January, 24–7.

Bynum, W.F. (1994) *Science and the Practice of Medicine in the Nineteenth Century*, Cambridge: Cambridge University Press.

Chapman, B. (1963) *British Government Observed*, London: Allen and Unwin.

Commission for Racial Equality (2001) *Racial Equality and NHS Trusts*, London: Commission for Racial Equality.

Coulter, A. and Ham, C. (2000) *The Global Challenge of Health Care Rationing*, Milton Keynes: Open University Press.

Dale, J. and Foster, P. (1986) *Feminists and State Welfare*, London: Routledge and Kegan Paul.

Davey, B., Gray, A. and Seale, C. (1995) *Health and Disease: A Reader*, 2nd edn, Buckingham: Open University Press.

Department of Health (1989a) *Working for Patients*, Cm 555, London: HMSO.

Department of Health (1989b) *Caring for People*, Cm 849, London: HMSO.

Department of Health (1990) *NHS and Community Care Act*, London: HMSO.

Department of Health (1991a) *The Health of the Nation: A Strategy for Health in England,* (Green Paper), Cm 1523, London: HMSO.

Department of Health (1991b) *The Patient's Charter*, London: HMSO.

Department of Health (1991c) *Press Release*, London: HMSO.

Department of Health (1992) *The Health of the Nation: A Strategy for Health in England*, Cm 1986, London: HMSO.

Department of Health (1994) *Being Heard: Report of a Review Committee on NHS Complaints Procedures* (The Wilson Committee), London: DoH.

Department of Health (1996a) *Choice and Opportunity*, Cm 3390, London: HMSO.

Department of Health (1996b) *The NHS: A Service with Ambitions*, Cm 3425, London: HMSO.

Department of Health (1997a) *NHS (Primary Care) Act*, London: HMSO.

Department of Health (1997b) *The New NHS, Modern and Dependable*, Cm 3807, London: HMSO.

Department of Health (1998) *Our Healthier Nation*, Cm 3854, London: HMSO.

Department of Health (1999) *Making A Difference*, London: TSO.

Department of Health (2000a) *NHS Hospital, Public Health Medicine and Community Health Service Medical and Dental Workforce Census, England, at 30 September 2000*. London: TSO.

Department of Health (2000b) *The NHS Plan*, Command Paper 4818, London: TSO.

DHSS (1973) *Report of the Committee on Hospital Complaints Procedures* (The Davies Report), London: HMSO.

DHSS (1976) *Prevention and Health: Everybody's Business: A Reassessment of Public and Personal Health*, London: HMSO.

DHSS (1977) *National Health Service Act*, London: HMSO.

DHSS (1980) *Report on the Working Group on Inequalities in Health*, London: DHSS.

DHSS (1981) *Care in Action. A Handbook of Policies and Priorities for the Health and Social Services*, London: HMSO.

DHSS (1983) *NHS Management Inquiry*, London: DHSS.

DHSS (1986a) *Primary Care: An Agenda for Discussion*, Cmnd 9771, London: HMSO.

DHSS (1986b) *Neighbourhood Nursing: A Focus for Care*, London: HMSO.

DHSS (1987) *Promoting Better Health: The Government's Programme for Improving Primary Health Care*, Cm 249, London: HMSO.

DHSS Circular HC(88)43 (1988) *Health Services Development: Resource Assumptions and Planning Guidelines*, July 1988.

Doyal, L. (1981) *The Political Economy of Health*, London: Pluto Press.

Ehrenreich, B. and English, D. (1983) *Witches, Midwives and Nurses: A History of Women Healers*, New York: Feminist Press at the City University of New York.

ESRC (1998) *Health Variations*, Issue One, January.

Etzioni, A. (1969) *The Semi-Professions and their Organization*, New York: Free Press.

Falconer, P. (1996) 'Charterism and consumerism' in R. Pyper (ed.) *Aspects of Accountability in the British System of Government*, London: Tudor Business Publishing.

Fitzpatrick, M. (2001) *The Tyranny of Health: Doctors and the Regulation of Lifestyle*, London: Routledge.

Flynn, N. (1993) *Public Sector Management*, 2nd edn, London: Harvester Wheatsheaf.

Flynn, N. (1997) *Public Sector Management*, 3rd edn, London: Prentice-Hall/Harvester Wheatsheaf.

Foster, P (1995) *Women and the Health Care Industry: An Unhealthy Relationship?*, Buckingham: Open University Press.

Fox, N.J. (1992) *The Social Meaning of Surgery*, Oxford: Oxford University Press.

Gabe, J., Calnan, M. and Bury, M. (eds) (1991) *The Sociology of the Health Service*, London: Routledge.

Garner, L. (1979) *The NHS: Your Money or Your Life*, Harmondsworth: Penguin.

Gathorne-Hardy, J. (1984) *Doctors*, London: Weidenfeld and Nicolson.

Gillam, S., Plamping, D., McLenahan, J., Harries, J. and Epstein, L. (1994) *Community-oriented Primary Care*, London: King's Fund.

Graham, H. (1984) *Women, Health and the Family*, Brighton: Harvester Press.

Graham, H. (1997) *Social Policy Association Newsletter*, Cambridge: Social Policy Association.

Grant, W. (1993) *The Politics of Economic Policy*, London: Harvester Wheatsheaf.

Griffiths, R. (1983) *NHS Management Inquiry*, London: HMSO.

Griffiths, R. (1988) *Community Care: Agenda for Action*, London: HMSO.

Griffiths, S. (1998) 'From health care to health', *British Medical Journal* vol. 316, no. 7126, pp. 300–1.

Ham, C. (1998a) 'Financing the NHS', *British Medical Journal* vol. 316, no. 7126, pp. 212–13.

Ham, C. (1998b) *Tragic Choices in Health Care*, London: King's Fund.

Ham, C. (1992) *Health Policy in Britain*, 3rd edn, London: Macmillan.

Ham, C. (1999) *Health Policy in Britain*, 4th edn, London: Macmillan.

Handy, C. (1985) *Understanding Organisations*, Harmondsworth: Penguin Books.

Hannagan,T. (1995) *Management: Concepts and Practices*, London: Pitman.

Harden, I. (1992) *The Contracting State*, Oxford: Oxford University Press.

Harris, R. (1995) *Enigma*, London: Hutchinson.

Health Departments (1989) *General Practice in the National Health Service: The 1990 Contract*, Health Departments.

Health Education Authority and King's Fund (1995a) *Black and Minority Ethnic Groups in England*, London: Health Education Authority and King Edward's Hospital Fund for London.

Health Education Authority and King's Fund (1995b) *Health, Race and Ethnicity*, London: Health Education Authority and King Edward's Hospital Fund for London.

Health Service Journal 22 February 1990, p. 294.

Healthy Sheffield (1985) *Our City Our Health: Framework for Action*, Healthy Sheffield.

Hennessy, P. (1992) *Never Again*, London: Jonathan Cape.

Higgins, J. (1988) *The Business of Medicine*, London: Macmillan.

Hudson, B. (1989) 'The elusive chimera', *Health Service Journal*, 19 January, 26–8.

Hughes, D. (1988) 'When nurse knows best', *Sociology of Health and Illness*, vol. 19, no. 1.

Hunter, D. (1993) *Desperately Seeking Solutions*, Harlow: Longman.

Hunter, D.J. (1993) 'The shifting agenda', in I. Tilley (ed.) *Managing the Internal Market*, London: Paul Chapman Publishing.

Iliffe, S. and Munroe, J. (1997) *Healthy Choices*, London: Lawrence and Wishart.

Illich, I. (1975) *Medical Nemesis: The Expropriation of Health*, London: Calder and Boyars.

Jack, L. (ed.) (1999) *Health and Personal Social Services Statistics for England*, The Government Statistical Service London: TSO.

Jones, L.J. (1994) *The Social Context of Health and Health Work*, London: Macmillan.

Joseph, M. (1994) *Sociology for Nursing and Health Care*, Cambridge: Polity Press.

Kandola, R. and Fullerton, J. (1994) *Managing the Mosaic: Diversity in Action*, London: Institute of Personnel and Development.

Karlsen, S. and Nazroo, J. (2000) 'The relationship between racism, social class and health among ethnic minority groups', *Health Variations*, Issue 5, January, pp. 8–9.

Kast, F.E. and Rosenzweig, J.E. (1985) *Organization and Management*, London: McGraw-Hill.

Katz, J., Peberdy, A. and Douglas, J. (eds) (1997) *Promoting Health: Knowledge and Practice*, London: Macmillan in association with The Open University.

Kendall, J. and Knapp, M. (1996) *The Voluntary Sector in the United Kingdom*, Manchester: Manchester University Press.

Kingdom, J. (1992) *No Such Thing As Society*, Buckingham: Open University Press.

Klein, R. (1995) *The New Politics of the NHS*, 3rd edn, London: Longman.

Klein, R (2001) 'Milburn's view of a new NHS', *British Medical Journal*, 322: 1078–9.

Law, I. (1996) *Racism, Ethnicity and Social Policy*, London: Prentice-Hall/Harvester Wheatsheaf.

Lawton, A. and Rose, A. (1994) *Organisation and Management in the Public Sector*, 2nd edn, London: Pitman.

Le Fanu, J. (1999) *The Rise and Fall of Modern Medicine*, London: Little, Brown and Company.

Le Grand, J. and Bartlett, W. (eds) (1993) *Quasi-Markets and Social Policy*, London: Macmillan.

Levitt, R., Wall, A., Appleby, J. (1995) *The Reorganised National Health Service*, 5th edn, London: Chapman and Hall.

Lindblom, C. (1959) 'The science of muddling through', *Public Administration Review*, vol. 19, no. 2, pp. 79–99.

Macdonald, J. (1993) *Primary Health Care: Medicine in its Place*, London: Earthscan Publicatios.

Macdonald, V. (1996) *Sunday Telegraph*, Focus, 14 April.

March, I. (ed.) (1996) *Making Sense of Society*, London: Longman.

Mayo, M. (1994) *Communities and Caring: The Mixed Economy of Welfare*, London: St. Martin's Press.

McKevitt, D. and Lawton, A. (1996) *Public Sector Management*, London: Sage Publications.

Meads, G. (1996) *A Primary Care-Led NHS*, London: Financial Times Healthcare.

Medical Services Review Committee [Porritt Report] (1962) *A Review of Medical Services in Great Britain*, London: Social Assay.

Milburn, A. (2001) Shifting the balance of power in the NHS, speech delivered on 25 April, http://intranet-qh/intranets/notice.nsf/vmain/8F5F2FA308A47E4.

Miles, A. (1991) *Women, Health and Medicine*, Buckingham: Open University Press.

Ministry of Health (1946) *The National Health Service Act*, London: HMSO.

Ministry of Health [Cranbrook Report] (1959) *Report of Maternity Services Committee*, London: HMSO.

Mishra, R. (1990) *The Welfare State in Capitalist Society*, New York: Harvester Wheatsheaf.

Mitchell, P. (1997) 'Rationing debate resurfaces in UK', *The Lancet*, vol. 350, no. 9072, p. 194.

Mitchell, R., Shaw, M. and Dorling, D. (2000) *Inequalities in Life and Death: What If Britain Were More Equal*, Bristol: The Policy Press.

Moon, G. and North, N. (2000) *Policy and Place: General Medical Practice in the UK*, Basingstoke: Macmillan.

Morgan, G. (1986) *Images of Organization*, London: Sage Publications.

Mullins, L.J. (1996) *Management and Organisational Behavior*, London: Pitman.

Naidoo, J. and Wills, J. (1994) *Health Promotion: Foundations for Practice*, London: Balliere Tindall.

Nazroo, J. (1997) *The Health of Britain's Ethnic Minorities*, London: Grantham Books, Policy Studies Institute.

New, B. (1996) 'Education and debate: the rationing agenda in the NHS', *British Medical Journal*, vol. 312, no. 7046, p. 22.

NHS Executive (1994) *Developing NHS Purchasing and GP Fundholding: Towards a Primary Care Led NHS*, Leeds: NHSE.

NHS Executive (1996) *Primary Care: The Future*, Leeds: NHS Executive.

NHS Women's Unit (1994) 'Career paths of NHS managers', *NHS News*, Issue No. 6, September, pp. 14–15.

Office of Health Economics (1990) *OHE Briefing*, London: Office of Health Economics.

Office of Health Economics (1997) *Compendium of Health Statistics*, 10th edn, London: Office of Health Economics.

Office of National Statistics (1997) *Health Inequalities – Decennial Supplement*, London: HMSO.

OHE (2000) *Compendium of Health Statistics*, London: Office of Health Economics.

O'Keefe, E., Ottewill, R. and Wall, A. (1992) *Community Health: Issues in Management*, Sunderland: Business Education Publishers Limited.

OPCS (Office of Population Censuses and Surveys), Social Survey Division (1992) *General Household Survey 1990*, London: HMSO.

Ottewill, R. and Wall, A. (1990) *The Growth and Development of the Community Health Services*, Sunderland: Business Education Publishers Limited.

Owen, B.G. (1990) 'France', in J.E. Kingdom (ed.) *The Civil Service in Liberal Democracies*, London: Routledge.

Parker, J. (1975) *Social Policy and Citizenship*, London: Macmillan.

Pascall, G. (1996) *Social Policy: A New Feminist Analysis*, London: Routledge.

Pencheon, D. (1998) 'NHS Direct: managing demand', *British Medical Journal*, vol. 316, no. 7126, 17 January, pp. 215–16.

Petchey, R. (1996) 'From stableboys to jockeys?', in M. May, E. Brundson and G. Craig (eds) *Social Policy Review 8*, London: Social Policy Association.

Peters, T.J. and Waterman, R.H. (1982) *In Search of Excellence*, London: Harpers and Row.

Pollock, A. (1997) 'Rationing in the "reformed" NHS', in S. Iliffe and J. Munro, *Healthy Choices: Future Options for the NHS*, London: Lawrence & Wishart.

Porter, R. (1997) *The Greatest Benefit to Mankind*, London: HarperCollins.

Powell, M. (1997) *Evaluating the National Health Service*, Buckingham: Open University Press.

Public Health Alliance (1988) *Beyond Acheson: An Agenda for the New Public Health*, London: Public Health Alliance.

Raleigh, V.S. and Kiri, V.A. (1997) 'Life expectancy in England: variations and trends by gender, health authority and level of deprivation', *Journal of Epidemiology and Community Health*, vol. 51, no. 6, December, pp. 649–58.

Ranade, W. (1997) *A Future for the NHS? Health Care for the Millennium*, 2nd edn, London: Longman.

Ranson, S. and Stewart, J. (1994) *Management for the Public Domain*, London: St. Martin's Press.

Rathfelder, M. (2000) 'Now inject some accountability', *Health Matters*, Issue 42, Autumn, pp. 12–13.

Rathwell, T. *et al.* (1995) *Tipping the Balance Towards Primary Health Care*, Hampshire: Avebury.

Reid, I. and Stratta, E. (1989) *Sex Differences in Britain*, Aldershot: Gower.

Research Unit in Health and Behavioural Change (1989) *Changing the Public Health*, Chichester: Wiley.

Rodmell, S. and Watt, A. (1987) *The Politics of Health Education: Raising the Issues*, London: Routledge and Kegan Paul.

Ross, R. and Schneider, R. (1992) *From Equality to Diversity: A Business Case for Equal Opportunities*, London: Pitman Publishing.

Royal Commission on the National Health Service (1979) *The Merrison Report*, Cmnd 7615, London: HMSO.

Scriven, A. and Orme, J. (eds) (2001) *Health Promotion: Professional Perspectives*, 2nd edn, Basingstoke: Palgrave in association with The Open University.

Sherrin, N. (1993) *In His Anecdotage*, London: Virgin Books.

Skellington, R. (1996) *'Race' in Britain Today*, 2nd edn, London: Sage Publications in Association with The Open University.

Small, N. (1989) *Politics and Planning in the National Health Service*, Buckingham: Open University Press.

Smith, L. (1987) 'Women and mental health', in J. Orr (ed.) *Women's Health in the Community*, Chichester: Wiley.

Stacey, M. (1988) *The Sociology of Health and Healing*, London: Unwin Hyman.

Straw, J. (1989) *Equal Opportunities: The Way Ahead*, London: IPM.

Tilley, I. (1993) *Managing the Internal Market*, London, Paul Chapman Publishing.

Timmins, N. (1996) *The Five Giants*, London: HarperCollins.

Towler, J. and Bramall, J. (1986) *Midwives in History and Society*, London: Croom Helm.

Townsend, P. and Davidson, N. (eds) (1988) *Inequalities in Health: The Black Report and The Health Divide*, Harmondsworth: Penguin.

Townsend, P., Davidson, N. and Whitehead, M. (1992) *Inequalities in Health: The Black Report and The Health Divide*, rev. edn, Harmondsworth: Penguin.

Ungerson, C. (1987) *Policy is Personal*, London: Tavistock.

Ungerson, C. (ed.) (1990) *Gender and Caring: Women and Welfare in Britain and Scandinavia* , London: Harvester Wheatsheaf.

Versluyen, M.C. (1980) 'Old wives tales? Women healers in English history', in C. Davies (ed.), *Rewriting Nursing History*, London: Croom Helm, pp. 175–99.

Victor, C. R. (1991) *Health and Health Care in Later Life*, Buckingham: Open University Press.

Vinten, G. (1992) 'Reviewing the current managerial ethos' in L. Willcocks and J. Harrow (eds) *Rediscovering Public Services Management*, London: McGraw-Hill.

Wakefield Health Authority (1997) *Partners in Health*, Wakefield: Wakefield Health Authority.

Walker, A. (1986) 'Community care: fact or fiction', in P. Wilmott (ed.) *The Debate About Community*, London: Policy Studies Institute.

Wall, A. (ed.) (1996) *Health Care Systems in Liberal Democracies*, London: Routledge.

Wall, A. and Owen, B. (1999) 'The doctors' dilemma: issues for a primary care led NHS', *Teaching Public Administration*, vol. XIX, no. 1, pp. 37–52.

Weatherall, M. W. (1996) 'Making medicine scientific: empiricism, rationality and quackery in mid-Victorian Britain', *Social History of Medicine*, vol. 9, no. 2, 175–94.

Webb, A. and Wistow, G. (1982) 'The personal social services: incrementalism, expediency or systematic social planning', in A. Walker (ed.) *Public Expenditure and Social Policy*, London: Heinemann.

Whitehead, M. (1987) *The Health Divide*, London: Health Education Council.

WHO (World Health Organization) (1978) *Alma Ata 1977: Primary Health Care*, Geneva: WHO/UNICEF.

WHO (World Health Organization) (1985) *Targets for Health for All: Targets in Support of the European Regional Strategy for Health for All*, Copenhagen: WHO Regional Office for Europe.

Wilkinson, R.C. (1996) *Unhealthy Societies: The Afflictions of Inequality*, London: Routledge.

Willcocks, A.J. (1967) *The Creation of the National Health Service*, London: Routledge and Kegan Paul.

Willcocks, L. and Harrow, J. (eds) (1992) *Rediscovering Public Services Management*, London: McGrawHill.

Williams, F. (1989) *Social Policy: A Critical Introduction*, Oxford: Polity Press.

Wistow, G. (1992) 'The National Health Service', in D. Marsh, and R.A.W. Rhodes (eds) *Implementing Thatcherite Policies*, Buckingham: Open University Press.

Wolfenden Committee (1978) *The Future of Voluntary Organisations*, London: Croom Helm.

Zola, I. K. (1972) 'Medicine as an institution of social control: the medicalising of society', *The Sociological Review*, no. 20, pp. 487–504.

Index